D0387683

SEX POINTS

SEX POINTS

Reclaim Your Sex Life with the
Revolutionary Multi-Point System

DR. BAT SHEVA MARCUS

hachette
BOOKS

New York

Hachette Go, an imprint of Hachette Books
Hachette Book Group
1290 Avenue of the Americas
New York, NY 10104
HachetteGo.com
Facebook.com/HachetteGo
Instagram.com/HachetteGo

First Edition: March 2021

Hachette Books is a division of Hachette Book Group, Inc.

The Hachette Go and Hachette Books name and logos are trademarks of Hachette Book Group, Inc.

The publisher is not responsible for websites (or their content) that are not owned by the publisher.

Print book interior design by Trish Wilkinson.

Library of Congress Control Number: 2020950738

ISBNs: 978-0-306-87387-4 (hardcover); 978-0-306-87389-8 (ebook)

Printed in the United States of America

LSC-C

Printing 1, 2021

To my clients,
who have taught me more than books ever could

CONTENTS

PART I

GETTING TO THE POINT

I'M BAT SHEVA—AND I CAN HELP

As a veteran sex therapist, I am frustrated almost daily by a persistent myth: that great sex comes naturally, and when it doesn't, there is something wrong.

Give me a break.

As human beings, our ability to love and be loved, and to desire one another, is a gift—a gift that takes work. Like exercise or eating right, it also takes practice and know-how. When women with common problems are dismissed, given shoddy medical advice, or simply not believed, they are being shut out from this amazing aspect of their life—needlessly.

If you've been told it's natural to lose your sex drive as you get older, or all you need is a glass of wine to relax, or it's all in your head, I want you to know your problems are fixable. If you're in pain, or are ashamed of your fantasies, or are thinking the sex should be good because you're young and in love, you shouldn't be. No matter who you are, I want you to know that you can have good sex. And I am here to help. *Sex Points* shares my hard-earned knowledge from years as a sex therapist. I am invested in your sex life—and I'm giving you permission to be invested as well.

Doctors don't suggest you talk through a broken ankle, drink a glass of wine for arthritis, or take a vacation for a rash. They diagnose and treat the problem. That is the same way it should be with problems having sex. When it comes to sexual health, commonsense practice seems to have gotten lost. Time and again, I find myself proposing solutions that the established medical system resists. A big part of the problem, of course, is that many don't take women's sexual problems seriously and dismiss or minimize them. Another problem is they barely talk about sex—at best, only 25 percent of medical practitioners do.

Good sex is possible for everyone, at every age, in every situation. And there's a solution for everyone. So, whether it's buying a "wedge" for your bed, using your most private fantasies to have an orgasm, visiting your partner in their office, using testosterone to get your mojo back, or injecting your vagina with Botox, if it's safe, I'll support you. That doesn't mean that once you hit on the problem, treatment is always smooth sailing. But just because sex isn't always easy, doesn't mean it has to be hard.

HOW THIS BOOK IS DIFFERENT FROM OTHER SEX BOOKS

Most books on how to have a good sex life focus on emotional intimacy, communication, and behavior—as if all your partner needed to do to fill you with desire was cover the bed in rose petals or do the dishes.

The truth is, while there are relationship and emotional components that are critical to a healthy sex life, for most women a hefty physiological or medical component is also driving their desire. In short, it doesn't matter how willing the mind is—the flesh would rather be doing the laundry.

We tend to think of a fulfilling sex life like a light switch—it's either on or off, and when it's off, we can only stumble around in the dark. But a sex life should be appreciated for the complex response it is, one that is made up of many different aspects of your life: age, home situation, hormone levels, relationship. These variables shift and change over time. Each can provide positive, experience-affirming value, or it can get in the way and drag down your sex life. Either way, all the elements and variables need to work together to make your sex life work.

Sex Points breaks down these variables in an easy-to-use point system—one that uses a threshold of 100 points for a healthy sex life. Each variable—such as pain threshold, or hormonal level, or emotional intimacy—has its own point value. The goal of this book is to help you find where you are missing points and give you resources for garnering new ones. You'll get a real live picture of your situation along with real live ways to fix things.

I KNOW WHAT YOU'RE GOING THROUGH

I am a fifty-eight-year-old sex therapist. I have worked with women and their sexual health issues for twenty years. I have six years of formal training and over eighteen being trained by my patients. I have a PhD in human sexuality and have published articles in peer-reviewed journals. I have been honored to be part of thousands of women's lives as they struggled to keep their sex life alive and passionate.

And when I was fifty-five, barely a year after my first hot flash, I lost my orgasms.

First, my desire took a nosedive. As sex drives are wont to do, it didn't disappear overnight. It was way subtler. There had always been periods when I really wasn't particularly interested in having sex, and periods when I actively didn't want to have sex. Hey, that's life. But those started becoming more frequent and lasting longer. And the times I actively *did* want to have sex seemed to be coming way less often.

As you can imagine, I wasn't happy about this. I fought it as hard as I could. (Come on, I'm a sex therapist!) I started meditating, making sex-dates with my husband, looking at sexy movies, using every trick in the book (and believe me, I know them all) to get back my mojo. But it wasn't helping—and it was so much darn work for something that, in the past, had been fun.

And then . . . then my orgasms started disappearing.

If there was one thing I could always count on, it was orgasms. They ranged from lovely to scream-from-the-hilltops, and they made sex more fun, exciting, and relaxing. Now? They were incredibly hard to have, and when I did, they were nearly nonexistent blips.

So, there I was, midlife, with almost no sex drive, hot flashes, and nonexistent orgasms.

I was pissed. But I was also grateful, because now I knew exactly what my patients had been telling me for years. Until now, I had been the dispassionate expert who could help them; now, I was living the experience—including the enraging way the world responds to a middle-aged woman who loses her sex drive or her orgasm.

Suddenly, I understood the rage women feel when the professionals tell them things like "It's just a different way of having sex. You should embrace the changes. It's time to move on to a different state of life, where cuddling is erotic."

Or when friends or medical practitioners suggest that women aren't paying enough attention or trying hard enough, as if, if they "just work harder at it," their sex life will go back to the way it was. As it is, we're good at blaming ourselves, and the women I see are turning themselves into pretzels trying to figure out what they are doing wrong or what they are not doing that is causing them to feel this way.

Or worse, when other experts and friends tell women that they must be remembering their old sex life wrong, or, even worse, that it was all in their head. That they weren't trying hard enough to relax, to make time, to appreciate their partner. That they weren't "working hard enough on themselves," or alternatively, on communication with their partner. That they must be harboring anger at their partner that was finally coming out. That they weren't embracing their body as it now was.

I knew those things weren't the case. And I knew how often during my sex life, my problems had been minimized, ignored, mismanaged. And I remembered how often I had faced problems and had no idea where to turn.

I started my marriage with painful intercourse that no one diagnosed. I lived through three pregnancies, one miscarriage, and a thirty-five-year marriage with a husband who has been on a complicated set of medications and who also lost his sex drive at one point. I have gone through great times in my marriage, and not-such-great times in my marriage. I have been on and off antidepressants and have lived through the resulting orgasm problems.

I have now lived many, if not all, of the complaints my patients come in with. And once you know, really know, what people are talking about, it changes everything.

For me, the driving force of my work has never been just an interest in the human body, but an all-consuming desire to help my patients, using whatever means necessary.

Early on in my practice, I got a phone call from a fifty-six-year-old woman whose pain during intercourse had been getting steadily worse for three years. She was resistant to coming in because she wanted to know exactly what we would do as treatment. She had already seen the three "top gynecologists in the city," and they hadn't been able to help. "Gynecologists keep throwing estrogen at me!" she said. I told her that, sadly, it was still very hard to diagnose and treat pain over the phone; reluctantly, she came in. Three weeks after beginning treatment, she was totally pain-free. "I don't know whether to laugh or to cry," she told me, "because it was such a ridiculously easy solution."

So, what had we done that the other providers in the city had missed?

Well, her doctors were right: she needed estrogen. But what they had failed to notice was that her vaginal muscles felt unusually tight, like those of someone who had never had intercourse.

I suggested dilators.

Our nurse practitioner, trained in traditional medicine, thought I was crazy. Dilators—a series of plastic rods inserted into the vagina to help with muscle relaxation—are typically used on young women who are having difficulty having sex for the first time. Nobody prescribes them for a postmenopausal woman who had been having pain-free sex for years. But all I knew was that we had a patient whose vaginal muscles felt tight to our nurse practitioner. Although dilators were usually used for younger women, it couldn't hurt to try.

In three weeks, the dilators had done the trick: her muscles had relaxed, and she and her husband were once again sharing the intimacy and love that comes from a satisfying sex life. But the reality of the situation hit home. How many other women out there are suffering from a problem with a "ridiculously easy solution"?

YOUR HAPPILY-EVER-FOR-A-WHILE

Your sex life is not static. It is an organic, ever-changing process. One day, you're a nervous bride who has chosen to stay a virgin for her wedding night. The next, you're eighty, and you haven't had an orgasm for a decade.

The important thing to remember is that each problem can be addressed and fixed.

Take a typical woman. When she embarks on her first sexual relationship, she might have tight muscle pain or a partner with premature ejaculation. Later, when she's pregnant, her libido may increase. But then, the kids are born, and she and her partner are fighting fatigue, and there seems to be no damn time for sex. The kids are banging on the door, and her ability to orgasm seems to collapse. When the kids become teenagers, they are up at all hours. By now, she's premenopausal, and her libido has taken a nosedive. Her husband's medication is making it difficult for him to maintain his erection. Once she fixes her libido, he doesn't seem particularly interested in sex and starts falling asleep in front of the TV.

I know this is not a pretty picture of the trajectory of our sex life. I remember going through these scenarios with a group of young second-year medical students I was addressing. I remember the horror in their eyes and then the uproarious laughter. But it's real. As I told them, our ability to maintain active fun sex throughout our life is predicated on our ability to move past the fairy tales of the media and to acknowledge this reality. Then, we can move on and find solutions for our patients.

This radical notion of sex as an ongoing project is difficult for even those of us who really work on our sex life. Recently, a former student named Rachel told me that some new problems had "cropped up" after we'd last seen each other. "It's probably time for that three-thousand-mile scheduled maintenance," I answered. "There is always something new that has to be addressed."

"I guess so," Rachel said wistfully. "But I feel like it shouldn't be that way for me."

I was stunned. I stared at the phone in my hand for a minute. "Rachel," I said. "We've talked about this so many times. There's never a happily ever after. There's only a happily-ever-for-a-while. For all of us."

When we say that our sex life should all flow smoothly after we get started having sex, what we are really saying is that all future sex problems are either because of an emotional failure in the relationship, or an unavoidable result of aging. But a joyful sex life is achieved through continual upkeep, attention, and effort. When you know there will be curve balls, you can anticipate problems, identify them early, and have confidence that there are solutions.

We all deserve a sex life that's fulfilling and satisfying. And good sex is worth fighting for.

OKAY. SO, WHAT'S A GOOD SEX LIFE?

Some people will want to have sex three times a day. Some, three times a month. But everyone wants to feel as though desire, arousal, and satisfaction are accessible. And, if the sex they are having is with a partner, they want their partner to feel good about it as well.

Whether it involves swinging from the chandeliers or simply a romp in the bed once a week, most people share the same goal. They want to *want*. That means they would like to prefer having sex to doing the laundry. And it means they want to be able to get turned on and engaged when they or their partner wants to have sex. And they want to get pleasure from the sexual experience and feel good and connected when it's over.

Sound simple, right? Unfortunately, it's not for many of us.

THE DOMINO EFFECT, OR "WHAT THE HELL IS ACTUALLY WRONG WITH ME?"

Often, women feel silly that they can't put their finger on the problem. That's because there's usually not one single problem, but a problem that has cascaded into a bad situation—one that has a mysterious source and seemingly no solution.

It might seem impossible to find a solution. But there *is* a solution, or more realistically a group of solutions, and you can have a healthy, fulfilling sex life. You just need to pinpoint the factors that are affecting you. And this book is going to help you do that.

Our sex life is a complicated interplay of body parts, emotions, and hormones. Physical health, personal history, experiences, beliefs, education, and confidence all play a role. It's easy for one part to break down and gum up the whole system. Finding that original problem might be trickier than you think. In addition, the ongoing problem may have created secondary problems. And sometimes these problems become a self-sustaining vortex.

Take a common example: avoiding sex and losing emotional intimacy. People get confused about which came first: are you not having sex with your partner because you need to work on your emotional intimacy, or is your emotional intimacy being affected by your avoiding having sex?

Another common experience: you might feel "stupid" and incompetent about sex because you have very limited experience, or are ashamed. Or you become ashamed because a simple physical issue is keeping you from enjoying sex. You could avoid sex because of a bad previous experience or trauma, or avoiding sex may be the cause of these bad experiences. You might have the hormonal profile of a ten-year-old, or crippling pain, and thus lack experience. And when you lack experience, it's hard to be confident.

How can you break it down? Here, I'm going to help.

THIS BOOK IS FOR YOU

Nearly every woman who comes to see me feels that she is somehow worse or different than other women. The most common question I get is "Am I normal?" So, let me make this easier. Yes, you are normal (whatever that means. I'm not quite sure). Yes, you probably have some unique challenges. We all do. But you are not that different, no matter what you think. And you deserve a happy fulfilling sex life. This book is for you.

It's hard to write a book that speaks to everyone all the time. At times, this book might seem as if it was written for someone else: sometimes the pronouns may feel off. Or sometimes the advice might seem to be meant for some other woman, in another situation. It seems that it's for someone heterosexual or partnered. You might feel it's not for you because you're transgender or gay. You might feel this book doesn't apply to you because you have a disability. Or are overweight. Or feel badly about your body. Or you have suffered from sexual abuse. Or are seriously depressed. Or you are single, or in a crummy relationship. Or, or, or.

Let me tell you this: *None* of my patients feels that they fit the mold. Everyone feels abnormal, or different, or beyond help, or that their problem has never been witnessed before in the history of time.

But, as I often like to tell my patients, "You're not that special. I mean you, *personally*, are very special, but your story . . . well, not so much."

No matter who you're attracted to or whatever type of relationship you're in (or not in), you will have many of some of the same problems. If you're single (you don't need a partner to have great sex); if you have a disability (your body may be different, or parts of your body may function differently, but you can have a satisfying sex life); if you are overweight and are used to being dismissed or ridiculed by your doctors; if you are gay, lesbian, or queer, in traditional or non-traditional relationships, this book can help.

I do want to specifically address those of you who have a history of sexual abuse and trauma, because I know how painful this is and that you may feel as if you will never heal from it or can never have a good sex life. I want you to know that I don't believe that is true! And I feel strongly that it is not helpful for a woman to believe that because she has a history of sexual abuse or trauma, she will not be able to have a full and satisfying sex life.

It is critical to understand that sexual abuse and sexual harassment affect women in different ways. I have seen a wide range of responses to trauma. This is why, when a new patient comes to my office, I take a full sexual history and always ask about sexual abuse. I want to explore how that abuse has affected her. When a woman reports something in her sexual history that is traumatic, or perhaps something that happened to her that could be categorized as sexual abuse but does not feel particularly traumatic to her, we have a conversation. I check in to see if the incident or situation has already been discussed with someone she trusts, processed, and looked at in the light of day. If it hasn't been, we set up dedicated time to talk about it and unpack it. We look at it together and see if either of us feels that it needs more processing. If need be, we'll set aside a few months for her to do some trauma work with a therapist. But at the same time, if possible, we start working on ways for her to move on and heal her current sex life. If she feels that she has faced the issue, has already talked it out, or that it is not significant to her current problem, we move on to a solution-based approach.

In almost every case, I tell women confidently that they absolutely can have a normal, healthy sex life. They should not feel trapped by their past or doomed to failure because of their history. If sexual abuse is in your history, you are not destined for a bad sex life. I promise.

You'll find stories from my practice throughout the book—women just like you who thought they were "the only one" with problems. I have changed all identifying details and in some cases have used composites. But rest assured, these stories are real, and I hope they help you see that you are not alone. Indeed, if it feels as though I am specifically describing your story, that is a testament to how universal some of our experiences are.

Ultimately, this book is for you, whoever you are. All of it won't be because we are all so different, but much of it will be. And using the point system should empower you to identify those parts and use them. The whole setup of this book is to help you look specifically for the places you are missing points and then choose your own adventure. You may need some modifications, but you're smart, you'll figure it out. Now, go get your missing points.

CHAPTER 2

GETTING TO THE POINT: 100

W hen I see a new patient, the first thing I do is listen to her story—and I listen well, because every story is unique. At the same time, I bracket her concerns and problems by categorizing them into different quadrants. Separating these pieces makes it clearer, so I can target my response. It also gives my patient a sense of relief, because the problem which seems so overwhelming has been broken down into manageable pieces. This gives her an idea of our goals, and the direction we're going to take.

As a tool to help me visualize and quantify the messy, disorganized, and often overwhelming analysis of a sex life, I use the model of a 100-point threshold. It's a concrete way for me to quantify and understand the contributing factors. I took this model from Michael Werner, MD, the medical director of our practice. He was using it to help explain to his patients the complicated mix of factors that are involved in infertility. It helped me appreciate how no one factor should be looked at independently. Helping my patients understand how different factors are involved and working with one another to create the problems they are experiencing has been invaluable. So, I created this tool to help you as well. When you start to use this model, you, too, will begin to recognize how your sex life is more than any one problem and is truly a sum of its pieces. You can get points from a huge variety of places: your relationship, your vacation, your hormones, your brain, your blood flow, your ability to focus. You can lose points from the same wide variety of places as well: lack of sleep, depression, no fantasy life, lack of hormones, lack of time, poor blood flow, kids, and laundry. ALL those things are important. When things are going well, and your sex life is humming along, you are probably living your sex life with a surfeit of points. In that case, when you find yourself having sex, even if you are exhausted, or under a lot of stress, it doesn't matter all that much because you have points to spare. It's when your point threshold is below 100 or even exactly at 100 that things get tricky.

It may sound silly to assign points to areas in your sex life. I totally get that. I also know that doing so has helped my patients understand a complex idea and has given them a framework for addressing problems in a more organized and less stressful way. Usually a patient comes in with the idea that "something" is broken or "off" or "low" or "not normal." Most women are thinking, "Do I not have enough hormones?" OR "Is my marriage a mess and I need a divorce?" OR "There has to be a cream that will fix my vagina." All of these neat, tidy, one-solution fixes would be great, if she were merely dealing with one very specific, very particular problem. And sometimes that is the case. But most of the times it isn't.

The day that I "got" the 100-point-threshold idea was the day that I turned a corner and was able to truly help patients. I was able to sit with a crying woman who loves her partner but saw the entire relationship starting to crumble because of a nonexistent sex life. I was able to encourage the newly married woman who didn't know how to "make things better." I was able to help them, and you will be able to help yourself, because you will get, really get, that there was no one thing that is "broken."

This 100-point system acknowledges that our problems don't have one source—but a solution (or several) may exist and we can approach problems from many different directions. This makes room for our sex life to be ever-changing, and for us to have a greater sense of how to control it when it goes awry.

So, if you are reading this book because "something is not right," I am going to help you stop thinking that "something" is one problem that needs a mysterious solution. Instead, we will look at each of these areas and figure out where you are missing points. Once you can see

those, I will offer you real-life solutions; I will help you navigate those
solutions to help garner some additional points until you've hit the
100-point-threshold and returned to—or finally gained—a healthy
sex life.

THE QUADRANTS

In my experience, nearly every sexual problem a woman has falls into
one or—commonly—more than one of the following areas:

PAIN, AROUSAL, ORGASM, DESIRE:

Here's a diagram that may make it easier for you to understand
the model.

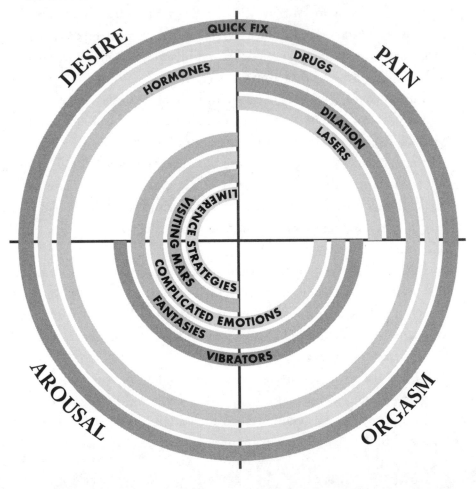

Let's go into some more detail about what each category entails (and if you don't identify with these right away, that's okay! The Sex Points assessment is coming up and that will help direct you):

Pain

> My vagina hurts.
> My vulva hurts.
> Intercourse hurts.
> Sometimes, the idea of the pain of intercourse is so scary, I can't even go there.

Arousal

> I think I want to have sex, but my body and/or my mind aren't on board.
> I don't get physically turned on.
> I can't seem to quiet that perpetual laundry list running in my head once I get going.

Orgasm

> I have never had an orgasm, or even gotten close.
> If I get close, I don't seem to be able to finish.
> I used to have orgasms, but they seem to have disappeared—and if I have them, they are pathetic echoes of what they used to be.

Desire

> I really am not very interested in having sex, even theoretically. Honestly, if my partner didn't care, I could go months, or even forever, without thinking about sex.

HOW POINTS CAN WORK

Here are some more examples of how to think about using the point system to help you. They will help clarify how different factors can become part of the equation.

Elise's Story _____

Take the hypothetical Elise. She's nineteen, so she's walking around with 90 points just from her hormone levels. That means she can pretty much have sex with anyone, anywhere, in any position, and it will be good. True, she's 10 points from 100, but since she doesn't have a lot of demands on her time and is starting to date in earnest, she won't have any trouble accumulating them.

Fast-forward four years. Elise is twenty-three, and she's met the man of her dreams. She is madly in love (+30 points) and the relationship is new and hot (+40 points). Well over her 100-point threshold, at 160 points, Elise is nearly always having great sex. She's happy as a lark.

Two years later, Elise is married to the man of her dreams. Although she loves him dearly, it's not so new anymore. She's also got a more demanding job, as well as more adult responsibilities. Still, she's got 120 points, which means their sex life is sizzling.

Now it's two years later. The first child arrives, then another. Suddenly, there are kids knocking at her door at all hours and climbing into bed (−20). By age thirty-three, her hormones have dropped (−20). Uh-oh. Elise is down to 80 points.

Now she rarely, if ever, initiates sex. It's hard to say yes when her husband approaches her. Her orgasms are few and far between, she is getting less aroused and lubricated. And she has no idea why.

At her next doctor's appointment, Elise raises the issue. The doctor hits Elise with this zinger: "How was your last vacation?" she asks. Elise tries to remember. "Our sex life was pretty good when we went to Cancún for the week," she muses. The doctor responds confidently. "If it's fine on vacation, it must mean it's psychological."

Elise leaves, but in a way, she feels worse than when she started. She knows that the sex was better because their vacation was different, exciting, calming. But she and her husband can't stay on vacation forever.

The good news for Elise is that sex was good on vacation because it gave 30 points, which means she wasn't that far below her 100-point threshold. She just has to figure out the best way to get back her points.

In our example, a drop in hormone levels was what brought Elise below the 100-point threshold. But the cause also could have been the onset of pain with intercourse. It could have been an ongoing tension with her husband. It could have been a lack of sleep. Loss of points can come from so many places, as can the addition of points.

But because Elise doesn't know she can get her points back, she starts to feel hopeless.

Cecile's Story

Cecile always had a great sex life. While she and her husband were dating, they had sex quite a lot. Unbeknownst to her, her **hormones** were fine, and her **relationship was solid and her husband often initiated sex.** She and her husband **always made time for sex** and she spent time (even not consciously) **thinking about sex,** watching sexy movies, buying herself great lingerie. They hit a rough patch when the **kids**

+70 points
+30 points

———————————
100 point threshold
+20 points

+15 points
———————————
total 135. They're good!

were little. **After all, they have 4 kids!** And there was a time when **the boredom and the sameness** just seemed to make her less interested with sex with her husband. They knew things weren't great but they made it a priority **to go away once or twice a year** and she noticed the sex always got better then. **Their regular sex life bounced back around the time her kids started high school.** Her relationship was pretty steady. They were having sex about once a week and sometimes it was fine and sometimes it was great. All things were good.

At age forty-eight, something changed. First of all, **intercourse started hurting** inexplicably. Her gynecologist said she couldn't see a problem, but every second or third time, it just plain hurt. On top of that, or because of that (Cecile couldn't really tell), she just found it harder to get her head into the game. Unbeknownst to her, her hormones had dropped as well, not terribly, but enough to make a difference. And she was avoiding sex as much as she could.

−20 points

−20 points

_____

Uh-oh. They're down to 95!

+20 points

_____

105. They're good!

+20 points

_____

125—good to go

−50 points

_____

down to 75

−20

_____

down to 55 UH-OH!

Lily's Story _____

Lily was twenty-three. She couldn't
remember a time she was interested
in sex. Her **hormones were nat-**   +60
urally okay, not great, just okay.
She grew up in a religious restricted
household. No one ever talked about
sex. She was a good girl and didn't
like to make waves. Without really
thinking about it, **Lily had shut
down her erotic brain**. She didn't   −30
flirt or put herself in any situations
where she could get turned on. Lily
was walking around with 30 points
and had no idea why anyone was
ever interested in sex! She felt like
she was crazy.
                                    _____
                                    30 points total

Miriam's Story (in Contrast to Lily's Story) _____

Miriam was also twenty-three.
She also grew up in a religious re-
strictive household, where almost
no one ever talked about sex. But
she was born **with a surfeit of
hormones**. And she had an older   +85
brother whose **sex magazines she**   +25
found at age twelve. She was really
curious about sex, even though she
couldn't have put it into words. She
was interested in boys and found

that they liked her back, which +20
was exciting. She even went so far
as to disobey her parents and climb
out the window a few times in high
school to meet up with her "boyfriend." She didn't understand how
Lily could be so uninterested in
something that seemed to domi-
nate her mind all the time.   _____

130

Here's where points can step in. When you're in tune with your body and situation, you can adjust your point profile as needed throughout your life. When your sex life is flagging, you can remember that everyone is different, but everyone can be helped. You don't have to be in a sizzling new relationship, or on vacation in Paris. You can reclaim ownership of your sex life whenever and wherever you need to.

Does that mean you need to be having wild sex every day to have what is considered a good sex life? Of course not. Only you can decide what constitutes a good sex life for you. For some people, it will be sex three times a week. For some, twice a month. Some people might want to walk around feeling frisky, whereas a lower profile might suit others. The most important thing to remember is you're in control. Once you know how to use points, if you experience a sexual problem, you can take a look at all the contributing factors and then figure out what to do about it.

Changes in women's bodies, lives, and relationships occur every day. It doesn't mean there's anything wrong with you or your partner, and it doesn't mean you're crazy. Some of these chapters break down the all-too-common and harmful attitudes many of us have toward sexuality. Others are about explaining what physical signs and potential problems we should look out for as we enter different life stages.

Sometimes that means a lot of clinical information about estrogen levels and the wonders of testosterone, and sometimes it includes tear-jerking stories from my practice.

Now that you have this book, you will be able to address those lost points no matter what causes them, and garner more in other ways. You'll know how to reach that 100-point threshold, and you will continue to enjoy the sex life you desire and deserve. Ideally, you want as many points as you can, because the higher above the threshold you are, the less you have to compensate for other losses.

So, let's look at each of the quadrants and discuss how you can determine whether you are missing points in that area, and how you can evaluate just how severe that point shortage might be. We'll also look at those factors that may cross over and affect more than one quadrant, and we'll talk about myths that get in the way of day-to-day sex.

Once you have the quadrants down, we will look at a whole host of potential solutions and ways to gain points in that quadrant. Many solutions you will be able to incorporate into your life with minimal effort and completely on your own. Some of these solutions may need a health-care professional to help you. But in those cases, having a deeper understanding of the problem and potential solutions will make all the difference. Once you are a critical medical consumer, you can become a true partner in your treatment, and save yourself a lot of time and heartache.

The first stop: a simple questionnaire to help you assess the points you have, or need, in the four quadrants. If the idea of a pencil-and-paper questionnaire isn't making you jump up and dance, or if like me you don't like to manually add, head off to my website to take the quiz electronically. I've set up a page just for you at www.SexPoints Book.com/Quiz.

CHAPTER 3

WHAT'S THE POINT?
OR READY, SET, SCORE

This questionnaire will help you home in on specific problem areas you may not realize are a problem. And when you see where the points are missing most significantly, you can get on the road to figuring out how and where to get more points. Note that some questions mention partners; if you don't have a partner currently, just answer the questions as best you can or score those answers "c" (3 points)

(To take the quiz online, got to www.SexPointsBook.com/Quiz.)

1. **During the last few months, how often have I had sexual thoughts, feelings, or fantasies either spontaneously or prompted by someone else or by something I read or watched?**
   a. I don't think I've had any.
   b. Maybe once or twice a month.
   c. About once or twice a week.
   d. Three or four times a week.
   e. Once or more times a day.

2. **During the past, when I tried to put something into my vagina:**
   a. No way I'm putting anything into my vagina.
   b. I wasn't able to get a penis, or anything else, into my vagina.
   c. I was only able to achieve partial penetration or penetration for a short time, mostly because of the pain.
   d. I achieved penetration every time, but once in a while it hurt a little. No big deal.
   e. Pain? Why should there be any pain?

3. **I can orgasm:**
   a. Not!
   b. If I work really, really hard at it with a strong vibrator and tons of concentration.
   c. If I fantasize or think about sexy things and stimulate my clitoris.
   d. Easily from a vibrator, sometimes from a hand or mouth.
   e. From almost anything, a penis, a hand, a mouth, a dildo, a vibrator.

4. **When my partner goes to bed and I know they are hoping I will be up there soon, I:**
   a. Am annoyed and feel pressured.
   b. Head over to the computer and work on some emails hoping they will fall asleep before I get there.
   c. Spend a minute finishing up what I'm doing and then start thinking about sex to get in the mood.
   d. Say "I'll be up in a minute" and mean it.
   e. Stop what I'm doing and hightail it up there.

5. **Over the past four weeks, I would rate my orgasms on a scale from 1 to 10, with 1 being nonexistent and 10 being explosive:**

6. **When I have sex with my partner or when I masturbate:**
   a. It's so frustrating because I never get aroused, wet, tingly, or excited.
   b. I am often anxious because sometimes I don't "stay" turned on and then it's a problem.
   c. I usually will stay aroused and lubricated for the whole time, and if not, lubricants or toys really help.
   d. I am pretty sure I'll be aroused and lubricated for the whole time.
   e. I know I will be aroused and lubricated and turned on pretty much until we finish.

7. **When I have sex (partnered or solo), I have orgasms:**
   a. Never!
   b. Maybe one time out of four or five.

  c. At least half the time we have sex.

  d. Most of the time we have sex, I end up having an orgasm.

  e. Every time!

8. **When I start fantasizing about sex:**

  a. Honestly . . . I don't fantasize.

  b. Fantasizing doesn't work at all for me. I don't get turned on.

  c. I usually can get turned on if I think about something sexy, but sometimes I have to work at it.

  • d. There are specific fantasies that really turn me on and I usually use them as my "go-to."

  e. I love to fantasize. It totally turns me on.

9. **What does intercourse feel like to me? Hmmm . . .**

  a. I actually don't have intercourse because, when I try to put something near or in my vagina, it kills!

  b. It often feels like ripping or burning. It's almost unbearable.

  c. I can take it or leave it. It definitely does not hurt.

  d. Intercourse feels good, most of the time.

  e. Intercourse is pleasurable and there is never pain.

10. **My favorite way to get myself in the mood is:**

  a. I don't like to try to turn myself on. It makes me uncomfortable and it doesn't usually work.

  b. I'm not sure what you are talking about.

  c. Sometimes I fantasize or think about sex, but I feel kind of foolish. I often just reach out to my partner.

  d. I like to watch or read erotica or think about another sexual encounter. That usually does the trick.

  e. I'm usually in the mood, so I can just start kissing or touching my partner and I'm good to go.

11. **When I tried recently to have an orgasm, either partnered or solo (stimulating my clitoris with a hand, mouth, or vibrator), I found that:**

  a. I really didn't try or I wasn't able to.

  b. It took a long time and was pretty difficult.

  c. Sometimes it was a little difficult but not really a big deal.

    d. A few times it was difficult, but the other times it seemed to be easier.

    e. No trouble at all. My orgasm shows up like clockwork.

12. **When I think about having sex with my partner (If you don't have a partner, no worries, score yourself a "c" [3 points] and move on),**

    a. I feel stressed out or resentful.

    b. I put it out of my mind because I'm too tired or overwhelmed.

    c. I smile and decide to think about it later. Sometimes I do. Sometimes I don't.

    d. I make a mental note to come back to that thought at a more practical moment and usually do.

    e. I consider telling them I'm in the mood or sending a sexy message.

13. **When I need to go to the gynecologist:**

    a. I have actually never been to a gynecologist. The idea is overwhelming and scary so I just avoid it.

    b. I hate going! There is so much pain and/or anxiety that I put it off as much as possible and really dread going.

    c. I just go. I don't love it, but I'm okay.

    d. I set up an appointment with someone I'm comfortable with and go. It's not really a big deal.

    e. I find the closest doctor on my plan and set up an appointment. I have absolutely no anxiety about it.

14. **During the past month, when my partner approached me for a sexual encounter:**

    a. I couldn't do it.

    b. I really didn't want to, but I did, and, if I'm honest, it was hard to get into it.

    c. I didn't particularly want to have sex, and hesitated a bit, but I decided to go for it and with a little effort on my part, it was fine.

    d. I hadn't really thought about having sex, but it was easy to go for it, and then it was smooth sailing.

    e. I was happy to have sex.

15. **Over the past few months, how often did I experience pain with vaginal intercourse?**
    a. I don't have intercourse because it's too scary and I know it's going to hurt.
    b. I try it once in a while and it hurts A LOT.
    c. Every once in a while it hurts a little, but it's no big deal really.
    d. There have been times in my life when intercourse hurt, but then it seemed to improve and honestly, I'm fine.
    e. Pain? No. I love the way intercourse feels.

16. **During the last four weeks, how difficult was it to reach orgasm when I self-stimulated (or had someone stimulating me) with a hand, mouth, or vibrator?**
    a. I didn't try.
    b. I wasn't able to achieve orgasm.
    c. It took a long time and was pretty difficult.
    d. Sometimes it was a little difficult but not a big deal.
    e. It was easy to have an orgasm every time.

17. **When I hear other women or the media talking about painful sex, I:**
    a. Want to cry because I know exactly what they are talking about.
    b. Wonder whether what I'm experiencing is what they are talking about. What they are describing is exactly what I'm experiencing.
    c. Know what that is like because even though I don't experience pain now, I have had times where intercourse hurt.
    d. Feel bad for the women who have painful sex.
    e. It's hard for me to empathize, because intercourse has always felt really good.

18. **During the last month, I guess I would describe my behavior this way:**
    a. I really avoid having sex with my partner or thinking about getting into a relationship because I really don't want to deal with the "sex thing."
    b. Pretty avoidant. I stay in the shower (or on the computer), hoping my partner will fall asleep before I come to bed or avoid getting too intimate in my relationships.

   c. I have sex (partnered or solo) pretty regularly, maybe three or four times a month.

   d. I don't have spontaneous urges to have sex, but when my partner approaches me, it's pretty easy to say yes and it's fun.

   e. I'm often the initiator with sex!

19. **When I have partnered sex or masturbate, on a scale of 1–10 with 1 being "not aroused" and 10 being "extremely aroused," I would say I'm a:**

20. **Let's talk about tampons. (If you are postmenopausal or don't get your period for any reason, just score this as a "c" [3 points] and skip this question.)**

   a. I can't imagine using a tampon. The idea is terrifying, and I know it will hurt a lot.

   b. I tried using tampons a few times. And it was a disaster. I don't think my body is built for tampons.

   c. The first time I used tampons, it was kind of uncomfortable, but I figured it out and it's usually fine now.

   d. I started using tampons when I was young, and after I started, I couldn't imagine going back to using pads.

   e. Why would anyone use anything besides a tampon or a menstrual cup?

21. **I start kissing or touching my partner or masturbating and:**

   a. I feel like nothing is happening and have to force myself to stay with the program.

   b. I work really hard to focus and get turned on. Otherwise my "to-do" list starts to intrude.

   c. My mind kind of wanders but if I breathe and focus I get turned on.

   d. I start feeling turned on pretty easily.

   e. I'm off, and ready to go!

22. **Let's talk about burning and itching around the vulva:**

   a. I have it all the time and it makes wearing certain clothing really uncomfortable.

   b. Sometime my vulva feels like it's on fire but that is usually only around my period.

   c. My vulva is almost never itchy or burny, unless I have a yeast infection.

   d. I've heard women talk about painful vulvas but I'm not really sure what they mean.

   e. My vulva is my best friend. She hasn't stung me once!

23. **The thought of having sex:**
    a. Frankly makes me a bit queasy.
    b. Seems a bit overwhelming and exhausting right now.
    c. Seems like a good idea and I tuck it away for later.
    d. Gets me turned on, and I enjoy the feeling for the moment.
    e. Gets me really turned on and I think about finding my partner or masturbating.

24. **If I decide to masturbate:**
    a. I can't imagine masturbating. Ever. It seems so weird.
    b. I have pretty much given up on masturbating because nothing ever happens.
    c. I don't do it often but I pretty much know what turns me on, so I pull out a book or video and can get going pretty easily.
    d. Sometimes I use a book, video, or audio to get into the mood and I am good to go.
    e. I usually don't need any outside help. My hands and my imagination get me turned on.

25. **When other women talk about how wonderful their orgasms are:**
    a. I am upset because I wish I, too, could have an orgasm.
    b. I get frustrated because mine seem so weak, almost nonexistent.
    c. I join in the conversation. My orgasms vary, but that's okay.
    d. I get it. I usually really enjoy my orgasms.
    e. I get competitive. Her orgasms can't possibly be as good as mine.

26. **When someone talks about "getting turned on":**
    a. I'm not really sure what they mean.
    b. I want to cry because my vulva and vagina feel like they went on vacation.

c. I think about it as a good way to get started having sex or masturbating.

d. I think about the things that turn me on: my fantasies, erotic books, and experimenting with my partner.

e. Just thinking about getting turned on, gets me turned on.

27. When I finish having partnered sex and it was good:

a. I am relieved that we did, and happy that I don't have to think about it for a while.

b. I tell myself to try and remember this so I won't be so hesitant next time.

c. I cuddle up and go to sleep happily.

d. I tuck the episode away for future fantasies.

e. I think, "Wow. That was great. Hope we get to do that again soon."

28. All the muscles down in my pelvic floor:

a. Seem to give me problems all the time. I have bowel problems, urinary problems, and pain with sex!

b. Seem to be kind of tight. I worry about sex and sometimes I have other pain.

c. Seem to work just fine. I rarely have urinary or bowel problems. Sex almost never hurts.

d. Seem to be working fine. I never have any problems.

e. Seem to be my friends. Sex feels great and I can even do splits.

29. When I have sex with my partner:

a. I get turned on pretty much never. It's really frustrating.

b. Sometimes I get turned on but it's not often and it's so much damn work.

c. I get turned on most times.

d. I almost always get turned on when I start having sex.

e. I get turned on really easily!

30. Having orgasms:

a. Seems like a mystery. I have no idea what that really means.

b. Is such hard work. It's just not worth the effort.

c. Is easier sometimes than others. I'm not sure why.

    d. Is pretty predictable.

    e. Easy as pie.

31. My orgasms have changed:

    a. Not at all. I have never had one.

    b. They used to be great. Now they are mere blips.

    c. Maybe they are a little bit slower to happen or weaker, but it's not a big deal.

    d. Not that I've noticed. They're fine.

    e. If anything, as I've gotten older they've changed for the better.

32. During the last month how often was I in the mood to have any type of sexual encounter with a partner? (It doesn't have to be intercourse.)

    a. If I'm honest, never.

    b. Maybe . . . once every two weeks, but maybe not.

    c. I'm pretty good to go at least once a week if they initiate.

    d. I like to have sex at least once a week.

    e. The more the better. I could have sex easily three times a week or more.

Scoring:

Give yourself the following points. For every:

    a. 1 point   c. 3 points   e. 5 points

    b. 2 points   d. 4 points

If the question is from 1 to 10, add your numerical answer.

LET'S TALLY

First, tally up all your answers. That should give you a quick snapshot of your overall sex life. The maximum number of points you could score, if everything in your life is perfect, would be 160. But that's going to be incredibly rare. If you scored over 100 points, chances are your sex life is working just fine. And if that's the case, good for you for getting this book because, as you know, your sex life is not static. One day, you may find your score dipping and then you have this book to address the issues.

If your score is below 100, all it means is that there is something to fix, and this book is intended for you.

If your score is way below 100, don't panic. It does not mean that you are beyond help. That's why I wrote this book. You are not alone, and things are fixable.

Now, I want you to go back and tally the questions for individual quadrants. This should show you where you are missing the most points. These scores will be your guide to this book and the chapters you need to focus on to gain points in those specific areas.

> **D. Get the total points** for questions 1, 4, 12, 14, 18, 23, 27, and 32.
>
> **A. Get the points total** for questions 6, 8, 10, 19, 21, 24, 26, and 29.
>
> **P. Get the points total** for questions 2, 9, 13, 15, 17, 20, 22, and 28.
>
> **O. Get the points total** for questions 3, 5, 7, 11, 16, 25, 30, and 31.

In a perfect world, if your sex life was humming along, each quadrant's score would total 32 to 40, leaving you with a healthy score of 128 to 160. But it's likely that you are now seeing low numbers across the board or some very lopsided numbers. That, my dear, is your key to figuring out where to go from here.

> Low numbers in D point to problems in the Desire Quadrant.
> Low numbers in A point to problems in the Arousal Quadrant.
> Low numbers in P point to problems in the Pain Quadrant.
> And, you guessed it, low numbers in O mean you need to work on the Orgasm Quadrant.

Now, there are two ways to use this book:

1. If your numbers are really lopsided—for instance, you scored a 35 in one quadrant and a 10 in another—you may want to dig into the chapters that describe the particular quadrant that's giving you the problem score. That should give you a more thorough understanding of the part of your sex life that is sorely missing points, and it will start to show you typical places where the breakdown occurs. It will guide you to those chapters that will be most helpful in gaining points in that quadrant.

2. If your numbers are low across the board, you may want to read through all the quadrants to get a better understanding of how and why your sex life is breaking down. Each quadrant's overview chapter also provides a guide to the subsequent chapters that will help you gain points in that particular area. Try not to panic. I really tried to make the chapters fun and amusing so you won't get weighed down with too much boring information.

A word of caution: Your sex life is not a chemistry experiment. These point guidelines are just that, guidelines. They are a way for you to take an overall snapshot of your sex life, as well as break down any problems you are having into manageable components and start addressing the individual parts that need attention. Approach it that way and it will help you best. You need points? Figure out where they are most missing and where they are most likely to come from. If one way of garnering points doesn't look like it will work for you, move ahead and look for alternative ways to get points into that quadrant. Don't drive yourself crazy with chasing 5 points here or there. Focus on addressing a variety of variables and concerns and incorporating solutions that will work best for you. Before you know it, you will be sailing right past that 100-point threshold.

So, let's dive right in, and *fix your sex life*!

PART II

UNDERSTANDING THE PROBLEM(S): THE FOUR QUADRANTS

CHAPTER 4

PAIN

*When You Wish It Were
Just a Headache*

> *— 30 to 80 points*
> *You may have lost some, or all, of your 45 points due to pain.*
> *Pain might also result in lost points in Arousal and Desire.*

Pain during vaginal intercourse can destroy your sex life. Period. After all, it's hard to have intercourse when you are afraid you're going to get clobbered over the head every time you become intimate. And second, while pain often impacts the other quadrants, it is less likely to be impacted *by* them. So, if you are having pain, it is critically important to address it first. If you are not having pain, go ahead and skip to the next quadrant, and at some future time, if you are having pain, know that this part of the book is here to help.

Some women have pain with sex all their life. For some, the pain starts after the birth of a child, or when there is a long time between relationships. Some have been having pain since they started having sex, and either were too embarrassed to ask for help, or didn't believe there was a solution. And for many, pain during sex starts inexplicably at any time, and they have no idea why it came, or what to do about it.

And friends and doctors aren't much help.

"Oh, we all have that problem."

"Try some Valium."

Or my personal favorite: "Just try to relax."

I've had patients quote their therapist's telling them that their vaginal pain was their "vagina's way of telling them that they 'weren't ready' to have sex." Oh, really? Or maybe it was actually their vagina telling them that it was time to find a new therapist. Or maybe, just maybe, it was their vagina's way of telling them that they were *in pain*. Sure, many sexual problems often include a mix of psychological and physiological factors, as do most things involving the body. But please don't let anyone tell you that the pain is "all in your head." All it means is that the doctor examining you can't see the problem or doesn't know how to address it.

One of the things that throws diagnosticians off when it comes to diagnosing and treating pain for women is that the types of pain and the causes can be so varied that, unless you are specifically trained to recognize and treat specific conditions, you can be easily fooled. Pain comes in many variations: itching, burning, sharp, dull, just at the opening, deep inside. And there are many factors that can contribute to vaginal pain: dryness, irritation, tightness, infections, dermatoses, involuntary muscle spasms, a bruised pubic bone, and small cuts or lacerations.

Also contributing to a difficulty in diagnosis is that the onset of pain can be gradual and subtle. Women have a hard time knowing exactly when the pain started! All they remember is that there *was* a time in the past when they had pain-free intercourse.

I'll hear things like:

"When Jonah was born, I remember it hurt a little, but then it seemed to get better. After Elyssa, I think things got worse . . . or maybe it was after Jenny . . . no, that can't be, because I remember having pretty good sex when we went to Greece on vacation. I don't know, maybe five years ago?"

And then I'll hear from women who *definitely* remember the onset of pain, because it was very sudden. There's an instance when they are having intercourse "just the way we always have, but it hurt so badly, and I made him pull out. And it hasn't been the same since!"

Your very real pain can be exacerbated by your fear and panic. Sometimes, pain makes a woman tense her body, or close off her mind to sex or her partner. It can be hard to treat the pain itself without also addressing the underlying or magnifying fear, and that is where therapy can come into play and can be extraordinarily useful.

Alternatively, your very real pain can cause other, secondary problems. If the pain has made you stop connecting sexually with your partner, then there is probably a great deal of anger or frustration on his or her side. If you feel that your partner isn't sympathetic or understanding about the pain, you may be furious. Sometimes when you stop connecting sexually, you feel, as many women say, "like roommates." When these secondary problems take on a life of their own, I've seen it undermine an entire sexual relationship. And, even when the pain has been addressed, those problems don't magically go away.

When pain has been affecting your sex life for a long time, you will likely have to address some of the personal and relationship problems that may have resulted from living with pain. But trying to solve the pain first is crucial.

You don't have to live with pain. Vaginal pain is treatable, except in the most unusual circumstances. Sometimes, you will need to search a bit to find the right physician. Sometimes, you might have to go to a few doctors or find a pelvic floor physical therapist. But don't allow yourself to get bamboozled into believing you have to live with pain and that the pain is in your head.

WHAT DOES VAGINAL PAIN LOOK LIKE?

Vaginal pain can be incredibly varied in its manifestations. However, for the most part it can be broken down into the following categories:

- You can't put a finger, a tampon, or a penis into your vagina.
- Going to the gynecologist for an internal exam is a scary and overwhelming prospect, and you may even take antianxiety medication to get through it.
- You can achieve vaginal intercourse, but it hurts.

- Your pain started when you started having intercourse and it really hasn't abated or changed much over the years.
- Vaginal intercourse hurts, but it didn't used to. Your vaginal pain started after switching medications or after a life change, such as the birth of a child, reaching menopause, or surgery or a trauma.
- You can achieve penetration, but when your partner goes deep, you have deep pain in your vagina.
- Your vulva (the area you see on the outside of the vagina) hurts, itches, or feels swollen all the time. Anything touching it irritates it, and you may find this gets worse or better continually.
- You think your pain may be age related, because it started when you were in your forties or fifties. You've heard other women talk about painful sex during menopause.

WHAT COULD BE CAUSING YOUR PAIN?

Let me make an interesting distinction here between types of vaginal and pelvic floor pain. There are conditions that affect your body and leave you with general pain in your pelvic floor, which are not particularly related to sex. You hurt all the time, either with deep pain or just plain ongoing pain. You bleed when you shouldn't. These pelvic floor conditions are the ones mostly commonly picked up by your ob-gyn and there is routine testing for them. So, if you are having pain, it truly is important that you start by getting things checked out with your gynecologist. They will be the ones to pick up what I'll call "standard" pelvic pain syndromes, such as contact dermatitis (a skin allergy), endometriosis (tissue growing outside your uterus), fibroids and cysts (bumpy growths in the uterus), inflammation (often caused by sexually transmitted infections).

However, if you are reading this part of the book, I'm guessing you have pain that hasn't been identified by your gynecologist and that is specifically associated with your sex life. And that can be uniquely frustrating and can leave you feeling as if you are running in circles.

This part of the book is intended specifically for you, to make you an educated, knowledgeable patient, who has a much better appreciation of your pain, why it might be overlooked, and what treatment options look like. Ironically, some of these pain syndromes don't necessarily require a physician to alleviate them, but some of them do; this chapter will help you identify the difference.

WHAT'S THE NAME OF YOUR PAIN?

When I give talks, I often joke that the names for these vulvar/vaginal conditions are getting harder and more difficult to say, and I wonder whether that is done in an attempt to discourage women from coming to ask for help. Dyspareunia, vaginismus, vulvodynia, vulvar vestibulodynia, genitourinary syndrome of menopause. Even physicians trip over the pronunciations and distinctions.

But these conditions are treatable and make the difference between a woman having a full and fulfilling sex life or avoiding sex completely. And unfortunately, these conditions, in my experience, are consistently misdiagnosed, overlooked, and left untreated.

The first term you will probably hear is **dyspareunia**, which means "vaginal pain with intercourse." Technically, all subsets of vaginal pain can be called dyspareunia. It's not a helpful diagnosis, though, because it doesn't suggest what the underlying condition may be. I remember working with one particular patient who had had ongoing pain for years. When we sent her out to another physician for a test, she came back triumphant. "I know what I have. He said I had dyspareunia!" Alas, I had to break it to her that all that meant was that she had a painful vagina and that we still needed to find the cause. So, feel free to diagnose yourself with dyspareunia.

Vaginismus is a pain condition whereby tightness of the vagina stops you from having penile penetration. It is also sometimes referred to as hypertonic pelvic floor dysfunction.

For some women, it feels impossible to get anything at all into their vagina. It can be so severe that it is impossible for anything to get in: a finger, a tampon, or a penis. For some women, penetration is possible, but it's incredibly painful. In many cases, vaginismus can be accompanied by a serious fear.

But, while I know it has a scary name, it's almost a slam-dunk in terms of fixing the problem. And in many cases, you might be able to solve this condition without the aid of a physician. This condition is so ubiquitous and so undertreated that I've dedicated an entire section to explaining it and outlining its treatment.

Vulvodynia is a condition of chronic vulvar pain at the entrance to the vagina. The location, constancy, and severity of the pain varies, but it is often described as burning, stinging, irritation, or rawness. There are many possible causes for vulvodynia and often this can be the hardest condition to treat.

Vestibulodynia or **vulvar vestibulitis** (See? I told you the names just get longer and longer) is a specific type of pain that often gets bundled into the diagnosis of "vulvodynia." It is pain in the vulvar vestibule, the small area of tissue just prior to the vaginal entrance. There are different types of vestibulodynia, and it is often difficult for a nonspecialist to determine what is contributing to the pain. The good news is that once an accurate determination has been made, vestibulodynia is treatable.

GSM is short for "genitourinary symptoms of menopause." Really? This is just a fancier way of saying the changes that happen because of menopause. Women in their midforties (perimenopause) and later, in their fifties, will often start to experience the symptoms of menopausal pain. The vagina will feel rough, raw or, in some cases, shut down, almost as if the vagina has disappeared. The tissue in the vagina may feel fragile, as if it is made of tissue paper, and it may bleed easily as well. This type of pain is usually quite easily and successfully treated.

WHAT CAUSES THESE CONDITIONS?

More interesting than the conditions themselves is understanding what causes the pain. Once you understand that, it makes it much easier to reach for a solution. So, let's run through the factors that are involved in all these conditions:

Hormonally mediated pain. Your vagina is hormonally ultra-sensitive. This means that the absence or change of hormones in your body will probably have a significant effect on your vaginal health. That can happen because of your age, as a result of childbirth, nursing, hormonal birth control, or other medication.

A classic example of women who have hormonally mediated pain are women who have gone on any hormonal birth control (the pill, the NuvaRing, Depo-Provera). Often, they find that their pain starts months, or sometimes years, after starting the drug. That's because these medications rely on changes in your body's hormone profile so as to avoid pregnancy. When the drugs lower your natural estrogen or testosterone, your vagina will sometimes be the first to know. More often than not, switching methods of birth control and using topical gels or creams that provide those hormones back to the body fixes the problem.

Another classic example of this are menopausal women. Unfortunately, as they hit menopause many, many women will feel like the invasion of the body snatchers has taken over their vagina. They may not be able to put it into words, but their lovely, reliable vagina *hurts*. It may have started off subtly and so they ignored it, but then the burning, irritated feeling just got worse and worse. As women go through the physiological changes both before menopause (perimenopause) and in menopause, the hormone balance in their body changes dramatically, and the vagina is the first part of their body to feel it. But hormonal problems can get compounded when muscles have tightened up. Which leads me to a second, be equally important, culprit . . .

Tight muscles. There will be a whole section of this chapter devoted to vaginismus, or tight muscles. When muscles are clenched as a result of pain or fear of pain, they can cause itching and burning on the outside of the vagina. I have had patients look at me like I'm crazy when I suggest that what feels to them like skin sensitivity or irritation is actually tight muscles. It doesn't make sense to them. So, to illustrate, I make a fist and clench as tight as I can. If I kept my hand clenched like this, I ask them, for hours, days, or even months, could you see how the skin on the outside would become red and hypersensitive? That's what is happening when your muscles are clenched for long periods of time. (If you think you are in that category, then the section that follows on vaginismus is for you.)

Lots of experiences can cause tight muscles. Childbirth, even from a caesarian section, can tighten up those muscles, as can an injury (one you were conscious of and even one you didn't notice) or aging. Hey, your muscles are tightening up in other parts of your body, why not also your vulva and vagina? Anyhow, in my opinion, these tight muscles, are the most often overlooked and underdiagnosed causes of pain, but they are imminently treatable and that is the good news.

Neuroproliferative pain. It's not extremely common, but nerve pain can develop from trauma, or as an allergic reaction to medication, or as a secondary result of nerve damage in other parts of the body. Even more uncommon, some women are born with an excess of nerve endings in the vulva. That means that there are just too many nerve endings in the area, or that the nerve endings are too sensitive and reactive. If that's the case, often surgery may be the only solution—and it's not an easy one. It's truly a tough surgery: When done properly, part of the vestibule is cut away and the tissue from the vaginal canal is pulled down and reattached. You can be on your back for six weeks and out of work for two months. But the good news is that the surgery has a 98 percent success rate. Recently, low-level cold lasers have also shown some promise in helping these cases. I'll talk more about this in the solution section, page 174.

THE BIGGEST CULPRIT ON THE BLOCK: VAGINISMUS

I'm guessing this may be the first time you've ever heard about vaginismus. It's not mentioned in those best-sex-ever stories that women's magazines are always running. Strikingly, nearly every woman who

I have ever met who suffers from severe vaginismus thinks she's the only one who's ever had it but the truth is, it's very common. Nearly 1 in 10 women suffer from vaginismus.[1] Women will live with this condition for years without talking to anyone about it, because they are so embarrassed. I'm guessing that's because no one else seems to talk about it and popular culture doesn't ever identify it.

Vaginismus is a condition whereby you have severe pain when you insert (or try to insert) anything into your vagina. Sometimes, there is a tremendous fear related to putting something in your vagina. Sometimes, there's no fear at all. But either way, it can be debilitating. Vaginismus, despite how rarely it is discussed, is incredibly common, can take many different forms, and is usually pretty easily treated.

What Does Vaginismus Look Like?

Here's how patients describe their experience with vaginismus:

"I was a virgin on my wedding night. I was also a virgin the next night and the next and the next. It literally felt like he was hitting a wall. After a few weeks, I sought help from my gynecologist. She gave me numbing cream. When the numbing cream wore off, I simply slipped out to the bathroom to cry."

"Sex was very painful. It was emotionally, psychologically, and physically hard to deal with; I didn't want to talk to anyone (other than my husband) about it. Part of me thought it would get better. Part of me was afraid to talk to my doctor about it. Part of me felt embarrassed—why couldn't I do something that everyone else could? I didn't even know how to go about addressing it. I felt like the problem was so big—I didn't know where to begin or what to do. It lasted for over a year before I sought help."

"For years, I put my feelings to the side, making excuses for why I could not use tampons or have sex. After being married for almost a year, my wonderful husband and I were still unable to consummate our marriage. Every time we attempted intercourse, it would end in tears and I could feel my confidence being eaten away. My husband is an incredible, understanding man, but I could see our troubles with intercourse affecting his confidence as well. There were no more excuses left to be made. Finally, I said enough is enough. I had to be fair to myself, my husband, and our relationship. I took my gynecologist's advice and saw a psychologist. Unfortunately, I left her office feeling more down on myself and alone than ever before."

"Shortly after going through menopause, I started experiencing searing pain during intercourse. I spoke to my gynecologist about it, and he prescribed some hormone cream. It didn't help the problem, and my doctor said there was nothing he could do. So, for many, many years, I abstained from intercourse with my husband."

I divide vaginismus into three categories:

1. **Primary—severe** refers to women who have really never been able to get anything into their vagina.
2. **Primary not-so-severe** are those women who have been able to get a penis into their vagina but have always had pain.
3. **Secondary** refers to those women who had a perfectly functional, pain-free sex life, and whose vagina, either subtly or immediately, goes on strike. Often, we see this with women who have just had babies or women who are perimenopausal or menopausal.

It's important to understand the difference between these categories. The treatment for those who have never had regular pain-free intercourse is different and much more straightforward than that for women who have had an ongoing working sex life yet who suddenly have unexpected pain. No matter which of the three categories sounds most like you, I encourage you to read all the vaginismus content that follows. It will help you better understand what's going on in your body, and also because it's so common, the more women who know about these conditions and can help other women, the better! Let's hear it for pain-sisterhood.

Primary Vaginismus (Both Severe and Not-So-Severe)

Primary vaginismus (or before-you've-ever-had sex vaginismus) can be scary and horrifying. Women with primary vaginismus feel as if they are hitting a brick wall every time they try to have intercourse.

Vaginismus lives on a continuum of the psychological and the physical: fear of pain, and actual pain. Almost all cases of vaginismus have both elements, but there is a huge range in one versus the other among women. So, we might see a woman whose muscles are tight but who isn't particularly fearful of penetration and can participate easily in the treatment. On the same day, we could see a woman whose muscles are not all that tight, but who is petrified of having something put into her vagina. Sometimes, we'll describe these patients as "table jumpers," because before we can even touch their vulva with anything, they are off the table and look like they are ready to run to Milwaukee—understandably!

Vaginismus can stem from simple causes: pain the first time a girl tried to put in a tampon or, when she first explored her body with her own finger, maybe she always just assumed something going into her vagina would be painful because she's actually never "seen" a hole there. Or—and this is most often the case—she just holds her anxiety in her vagina. Some women tense their back or neck. Some women tense their vaginal muscles without realizing it, and those muscles become extremely tight over time. One of the most frustrating things for women who have primary vaginismus is that people assume that it must have its roots in childhood sexual abuse. But that is simply not the case.

Here's the analogy I use to describe primary-severe vaginismus when I am lecturing to psychologists and even physicians. "What might your reaction be if I told you I was going to put a pen into your eye? If I said, 'Listen, your pupil is actually a hole. Not to worry. It won't hurt a bit. It might actually feel good.' You would look at me as though I had three heads and run for your life."

My patients with severe vaginismus feel that way when they try to have sex—or even go on the examination table. And that makes inserting anything as a course of treatment difficult. Often teaching these women to relax their muscles and learn to stretch these muscles is overwhelming emotionally and we have to work with antianxiety medications, behavior modification, and relaxation exercises.

It's hard to point to one characteristic in women who present with vaginismus. Vaginismus patients are often what would be described as type A personalities: tense or anxious and very used to taking charge of their life, being productive, getting a lot done. As you can imagine, this can make things worse, since their body is not responding to them, or doing what they think it should! Many vaginismus patients have other phobias. They may have a fear of heights—or flying, driving, or even needles.

Vaginismus patients often compartmentalize. They decide not to think about the problem because they feel so hopeless and out of control when they do. They and their partners may also start to avoid sex altogether. Every time they try, it hurts, or they fail again. Some feel so terrible about the situation, they find it easier not to think about it, and not having sex at all is one way to do that. Or, if they are single, they avoid dating.

It's also important to remember that although vaginismus can have an impact on you at almost any stage of your sex life—when you are starting your sex life, immediately after you have children, or even as you head into menopause—primary vaginismus can impact you more broadly because of the overwhelming fear. We often see patients who have waited years to seek treatment and are only finally doing so because their marriage is in crisis. Single women may even go so far as to stop dating altogether because they know at some point sex will rear its head. I've had more patients than I can count who have never dated and had every excuse in the book as to why not—but what it really came down to was that they felt that there was something significantly wrong with them. In their mind, they were destined to be alone.

Here's the deal. You really can have a great sex life even if you have vaginismus. There are dozens of ways to have sex that don't involve putting a penis in the vagina: oral sex and anal sex and manual sex, and feathers and breasts and stomachs and asses. Sometimes we see vaginismus patients who haven't let it get in the way of their sex life. They maintained a fun, regular sex life without intercourse. But more often than not, the fear and stigma get to be too painful, and women shut down their sex life altogether.

Secondary Vaginismus

If your vaginismus is not so severe or it's secondary (you've had years of nonpainful intercourse), the treatment is faster, easier, and less complicated. You can get something into your vagina and the idea doesn't fill you with dread and panic. In this case, your job is to work through the muscle contractions. You will slowly learn to stretch your muscles while relaxing your pelvic floor. It's a slow process but not overwhelming or extremely painful. It's just a matter of doing daily exercises and can often be treated in four to eight weeks depending on how tight the muscles are. And for you, if there is not a lot of fear, you can probably do most of your treatments by yourself, without much professional guidance. You can get started at home.

How Is Vaginismus Treated?

The muscles in your vagina should essentially work like a turtleneck sweater. When something (a penis, a finger, a tampon) pushes through your vagina, your vagina should easily expand, and when something pulls out, it should revert to its original size. Treating vaginismus, whether it's primary or secondary, means you have to train the muscles to relax and stretch. The treatment is simple: You use vaginal dilators (which is just a fancy word for "stretcher") to gradually teach the muscles to relax and stretch or restretch.

Vaginal dilators are instruments that are developed specifically for use in the vagina. Essentially, they are varying sizes of tubular sticks, which can be made out of plastic, silicone, or shatterproof glass. They are fairly inexpensive, easily accessible, and perhaps the most useful item in our toolkit. The ones we use in our practice are hefty plastic, and come in eight sizes. Starting with a stick about the diameter of your pinkie (the extra-small), the patient uses a slightly wider dilator until it is the size of an average penis, and up to a Polish kielbasa.

The goal with dilation is to retrain the tight vaginal muscle to respond differently to the anticipation of penetration. Slow, systematic, progressive dilation will help you connect your body and your mind, so you don't have unconscious clenching of the vagina. We use dilation for women who are afraid of having intercourse for the first time, are experiencing pain after childbirth, are dating partners with a large penis, are heading into menopause, or have gone through menopause.

If you think that working with dilation is right for you, later in this book (Chapter 12), I'll give you guidance on using dilators either by yourself or with a medical practitioner, as well as pinpointing some of the classic stumbling blocks. Not only will you find some ideas about how to manage your anxiety, you'll find some sympathy with how hard this can be to do. You need to trust that there is a way to treat your vaginismus, that you are not alone, that there truly is a solution.

"WHAT IF I REALLY, REALLY CAN'T DO IT?"

I will never forget Emily. After weeks of trying to insert dilators, using deep breathing, antianxiety medication, and hyperventilating in our office, she sat up on the exam table and said, "Bat Sheva, there must be another way!" I felt awful for Emily, because I didn't have another way at a time. But I kept my eyes and ears open and I set out to find a treatment method for those women who are overwhelmed, fearful, and panicked, and for those with a significant history of pain or those who have not been successful using traditional dilator therapy.

Not long afterward, I found the answer from an ingenious plastic surgeon in New Hampshire, Peter Pacik.[2] The answer was Botox. Yes, Botox! The very same neurotoxin that people inject into their forehead and around their eyes to erase wrinkles. Botox works by blocking the chemical that sends a message to your brain to tense a muscle. If you try to frown, the muscles won't tense. It works the same way in your vagina! Even if you are scared, your vagina won't tense up. And that takes much of the fear and distress out of the first few steps of treatment.

Here's how it works: The woman is put under conscious sedation for a short period of time. The doctor massages the introital muscles to break the muscle spasms and injects Botox and a topical anesthetic in the vaginal walls. Finally, the physician inserts a large dilator.

The patient wakes up with the large dilator inside her—something most patients could not imagine ever happening to them. It's scary, but it's also very liberating.

This is a tremendously helpful first step to achieving pain and worry-free penetration, but it is only a first step. I'm always careful to emphasize that the Botox procedure does not solve the problem. It's not a cure-all, but a crucial breakthrough. Your brain still needs to learn to communicate with your vagina. Once the procedure is over, you still need to learn to insert the dilators yourself, feel comfortable with touching your vulva and vagina, and relax with penetration. This is when the real work begins. You learn how to get comfortable with the idea of inserting something into your vagina, internalize the idea that there is really no pain, and then make the transfer to intercourse. If you want to pursue this course of treatment, take a look at Chapter 12.

Two Different Vaginismus Stories

KATIE'S STORY (PRIMARY VAGINISMUS)

I'll never forget the way Katie looked at me, her eyes brimming with tears, as she confided: "My sister and two of my best friends are expecting babies. I am so happy for them . . . or at least I'm trying to be. But I want a baby so badly. I'm trying not to think only about myself, really, I am. I am making baby showers and taking them to doctor's appointments but it's just so hard . . . " Her voice broke and the tears came down in earnest.

Katie still hadn't given up sex entirely. She and her husband, Mitch, had figured out other ways to give pleasure to each other and they were doing so occasionally. This was one of the most important points of strength for this couple. They still felt connected. But Katie's inability to have children was a persistent source of misery.

Katie was so scared of penetration that when we tried to examine her, she pushed her thighs together and edged off the table. But she was also very clear that she wanted to tackle the problem head on. So, after explaining the situation and treatment, we used that exam to help Katie put in the first dilator.

Like many primary vaginismus patients, Katie was really scared—she trembled a little, and had to pause—many times (which we did). We walked her through some guided breathing exercises until Katie felt ready to try. The dilator did hurt, but once it was inside, the burning sensation and sense of strangeness began to ease a little bit.

Getting that first small dilator was a huge victory. It meant that Katie was able to overcome her fear of penetration enough to get to work.

We sent Katie home from that first visit with her first dilator and a homework assignment. Her job was to use the small dilator daily for ten minutes. However scared or uncomfortable she felt about the dilation process, she had never been one to shirk her homework. Katie used those dilators every day, while she lay on her bed with the dilator in place, book in hand, or watching TV. Each time, she experienced burning discomfort, but as she stuck with it, it became easier. Gradually, she learned how to tolerate this alien presence in her body.

During the course of the next two months, Katie would come to our office once a week. Each week, we would introduce a slightly larger dilator. Some weeks, she'd move up in dilator size. Some weeks, she wouldn't feel ready. After each session, she would sit down with me to talk over the emotions that she was experiencing.

The weight that Katie had been carrying for nearly ten years was beginning to lift, along with her sense of isolation and shame. This problem was no longer a wordless thing that she and her husband, Mitch, kept as a mutual secret. It had a name. Other couples had suffered from it. And there were practical tools they could use to deal with it.

Two months after that first visit, Mitch and Katie had intercourse for the first time. The moment Mitch penetrated her shocked Katie with its intensity. As he moved inside her, she felt free. It was as though she and her husband had finally crashed through the wall that they had slammed into over and over again.

Several weeks later, Katie woke early one Sunday morning with an excited sense of possibility. She was sitting on her couch at 5:30 a.m. as the two lines slowly formed on a pregnancy kit stick. Katie showed up with sparkling eyes and flowers for me. Katie had blossomed in the four months we had known her. She seemed to stand taller, smile bigger, and walk with newfound confidence. I can't tell you how thrilled I was when nine months later, I received a picture of a beautiful baby boy.

JOANIE'S STORY (SEVERE VAGINISMUS)

When Joanie came to see me, she was crying so hard the minute she sat down that she could barely get any words out. On her medical forms, under the heading of, "Please tell us what brings you here today" she wrote: "Unable to have sex."

"You're feeling pretty hopeless right now?" I asked, even though the answer is obvious.

"We've been married almost four years. I've seen three different gynecologists. We've seen a general therapist and a sex therapist. No one can help us."

And she told me her story.

Joanie and her husband decided to hold off on intercourse until they were married. At that time, they had a great non-intercourse-based sex life, using hands and mouth to give each other pleasure. Nearly every time they were together, they would be sexually active, and they both found it fun and exciting.

Once they got married, their sexual activity focused on intercourse. At first, they weren't frustrated by their difficulty. They had assumed that as newlyweds, it might take a while for them to achieve penetration.

But as the months dragged on and Joanie's pain continued, sex started to be a chore rather than a pleasure. She would feel awful about herself, broken and "abnormal." Her husband would feel hopeless and confused. He started having a difficult time keeping his erection. Sex was no longer fun. Eventually, they stopped trying to have intercourse and, at the same time, stopped having any type of sex. Their sex life dwindled to nothing.

By the time Joanie came to see me, they had gone for almost six months with no sexual contact. This had taken a toll on the relationship.

Joanie couldn't get the dilators in no matter how calmly and gently we worked with her. Breathing exercises and Valium didn't help. She was panicky that this would never get better. After a month of therapy sessions, we talked about the idea of using Botox injections. She scheduled her appointment for two months down the line. In the meantime, she continued to come in for talk therapy and I encouraged her to get back to having (nonintercourse) sex at least once a week with her husband. Just knowing there was a solution, and by regularly reconnecting with her husband, she already looked brighter. She was hopeful.

On a sunny Monday morning, she came into our surgical center, filled out some paperwork, and was put under conscious sedation.

Waking from the anesthesia, Joanie was still a bit groggy. "Are you done?" She asked. Melissa, our nurse practitioner, nodded. "NO way! Am I . . . am I okay?" She asked. "Is everything okay down there?" "Everything is great. And you have the largest dilator in right now, as we speak," Melissa said. "Really???" Joanie reached down and touched the dilator coming out of her vagina. "I don't feel it. At all."

For the next hour or so, Melissa sat with Joanie and helped her move the dilator in and out. Because of the lidocaine Joanie felt no pain. Within the next three to four days, the Botox would make it impossible for her to tighten her muscles. Joanie went home that day, slept with the dilator and returned the next day. She was exultant. "I can do this!!" We saw Joanie a few more times, helped her get more and more comfortable with dilating and then, when she was ready, met with her and her husband and gave them instructions on how to go about having intercourse for the first time.

Joanie checks in from time to time with us. Her sex life is back on track.

VULVODYNIA AND VESTIBULODYNIA

These conditions are often mixed up, misunderstood, and more often than not, misdiagnosed or mistreated. That's why it's key that you educate yourself so you can identify what you think you might have. You should be able to describe and outline your situation to a physician and, this is critical, you should be able to tell whether the physician you are speaking to is knowledgeable enough to treat you.

Vulvodynia is a condition of chronic vulvar pain that lasts for at least three months. When we say "the vulvar region," I'm including the pad of fatty tissue at the base of your abdomen (if you want the official name, it's the mons pubis), the labia (the flaps of skin around your vulva), the clitoris, and the vaginal opening. Most patients describe the pain as burning, stinging, irritation, or rawness.

Part of what makes it difficult to diagnose vulvodynia is that it can vary significantly from woman to woman:

- There are women who have it "localized" (affecting a specific area of the vulva) and there are those who have it "generalized" (throughout the entire vulva) or mixed (localized and generalized).
- Some women have pain all the time. More commonly, women only have it sometimes, either certain times of the month or the pain is what we call "provoked" (pain occurring with contact or attempted vaginal penetration) or spontaneous (pain occurring without external stimulus). Sometimes, you guessed it, the pain is mixed (provoked and spontaneous).
- For some women the pain is primary (pain has always been present), but for significantly more women, the pain is secondary (at one time the patient was pain-free, but now the pain has developed).
- Women also experience the pain in different ways: intermittent, persistent, constant, immediate, delayed.

Vestibulodynia is a subset of vulvodynia. You may also hear the term *vulvar vestibulitis*. They tend to get used interchangeably. *Vulvodynia* refers to any pain in the vulva. *Vestibulodynia* is describing pain in response to pressure *specifically at the vulvar vestibule (the ring of tissue surrounding the vaginal opening)*. Often, you can see actual redness of the vulvar vestibule. Usually women only feel this pain when they are trying to put something into the vagina, such as a tampon or while having intercourse.

A physician will usually diagnose vulvodynia and vestibulodynia by taking a full history of the pain and doing a genital exam. The genital exam will include the "swab test," whereby the clinician will examine and press the spot on your vulva and vestibule with a moistened swab to identify where you might be feeling pain. They will also test your pelvic floor muscles to see whether they are tight as well. It's likely they will take cultures to rule out infections.

There are multiple causes of vulvodynia and vestibulodynia. They are the same as I outlined in the beginning of this chapter (pages 42–44), but as a review:

- Hormone fluctuations. These can be the result of childbirth, breastfeeding, birth control, other medications, or menopause.
- Pelvic floor dysfunction (high pelvic muscle tone and tight muscles)
- Increased production of nerve endings in the vestibule (congenital or acquired)
- Vaginal infections
- Contact or allergic irritants

Vulvodynia treatment varies depending on the underlying cause. This is why careful examination and correct diagnosis is so important. Treatment can include hormonal creams, medication changes, vaginal dilation, pelvic floor physical therapy, muscle relaxant suppositories, treatment for underlying infections, vulvar hygiene changes, vaginal injections under anesthesia, and surgery. Chapter 12 offers more direction on many of these treatments. I would also suggest you look carefully at Chapters 9–11 to see whether medications, be they creams and pills, might be either helping or making things worse.

What many people don't get is that, like other chronic pain sufferers, vulvodynia patients can get frustrated, depressed, demoralized, and can begin to feel hopeless. Because it is so often misdiagnosed and misunderstood, women start to feel that they will never find a solution and they will have to live with pain for the rest of their life.

If you are facing one of these conditions, you might want to consider working with a therapist who can support you emotionally during your search for help. It is not that emotional or mental health issues have caused these problems; rather, getting emotional and psychological support can be extremely helpful when dealing with any long-term pain, and these conditions have a way of deeply affecting how women feel about themselves as women, as sexual beings, and as partners.

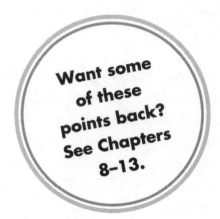

Want some of these points back? See Chapters 8–13.

CHAPTER 5

AROUSAL

The Agony of No Ecstasy

> *— 30 to 60 points*
>
> *You may have lost some, or all, of your arousal points.*
>
> *Problems with arousal may also have led to lost points in desire and orgasm.*

Look back and try to remember the first time you ever got turned on. Was it when you stumbled across "sexy" magazines or books that belonged to your parents? Was it on a school trip when a boy said something to you unexpectedly on a bus? Was it watching a TV show and seeing two people kissing? It felt good, it felt weird, it felt secret, it felt wrong, but it *felt*.

Now, you want to have sex. You really do. You've been thinking about it, planning it, and maybe even counting on it. But then when the time comes, it feels like your body has gone on strike. You don't get that butterfly feeling in your stomach. You don't feel tingly or turned on. You are not getting wet like you once did.

And your head? Somehow it is hard to keep it on task. You're thinking of your to-do list, a TV show plot, or a conversation you had with your girlfriend. Eventually, it starts to feel like so much work to stay focused on the sex that you start wondering whether it's even worth it.

What's wrong? Well, I'd say you have an arousal problem.

When you're aroused, your genitals feel warm and tingly, they lubricate or "get wet." Some women talk about getting so wet that they "drip" or "cream" their underwear. Some women simply feel something happening in their genital region. Their heart rate and respiration changes. Some fantasize. For most women it is a pleasurable experience—very visceral, very much from their depth of being.

Our hormones prime our body to be erotic and to feel erotic. We get turned on and something fun and fluttery goes on in our body.

But if the part of your brain that says, "Hey, this feels really good," never kicks in, it can feel mechanical—even disgusting.

Without arousal, sex can seem as yucky as it did before puberty.

PROBLEMS WITH AROUSAL

Problems with arousal can be difficult to identify because arousal is just plain confusing. You may be able to get aroused sometimes, or, if you put a whole lot of mental effort into it, you can get going. Because it seems somewhat under your control, you can get angry at yourself or frustrated. You believe you're not trying hard enough or just not pushing the right buttons.

Instead, let's think of arousal as the first step up the ladder of sex. You may search around for other usable footholds. You try the bottom shelf of a bookcase, but it starts to fall over. You might try jumping up to grab the object. But nothing works well. Where is the bottom rung of the stepladder? As the arousal gets harder and harder to access, the next rung of the ladder seems more and more unreachable, until at some point it is so far out of your line of vision, it just doesn't exist.

AROUSAL AND DESIRE ARE NOT THE SAME!

I hope this is one of those times when this book gives you an aha! moment. Too often, in sexual health, arousal and desire are mixed up. Patients do it all the time. They come in, drop down at my table, and sigh loudly. "I have no desire!" But then, when I start to ask questions, what I find out is that they do actually have desire. They want to have sex. Sometimes they even plan longingly for it. But then, when they start having sex, nothing happens. They don't get turned on. Their brain just goes off on its own tangent, or their body feels like it's taking a nap. That is not a desire problem. That is an arousal problem. And the sooner we acknowledge that there are two individual components of a woman's sex life, the sooner we can get on our way to fixing the problem.

Here's the deal. There are women who don't get turned on, despite wanting to have sex. Sometimes, they ultimately stop wanting to have sex, but that is not because they don't have desire; rather, every time they actually start to have sex, it's such a miserable disappointment. Similarly, I work with women who have zero desire to have sex. They have to drag themselves into the bedroom despite the fact that they get turned on easily, have orgasms, and enjoy the sex! I literally had a huge argument with a male specialist in the field who insisted there was no such thing. It's not possible, he said, that a woman gets turned on, enjoys sex, and then is completely uninterested afterward. Really? Well, I have news for you. Not only do these women exist, we see them every week.

I think it is critically important for a woman to learn for herself how to understand and distinguish between these two quadrants. Once you can define your problem, it should make finding solutions easier and more straightforward. It will also give you a better idea of what your "end goal" or success will look like.

WHAT DO AROUSAL PROBLEMS LOOK LIKE?

Here's how women with arousal problems generally describe their experience:

- I never ever get turned on anymore when we're having sex. I have to pretend to be interested!

- I can get turned on when I'm having sex, but it is just so much darn work.
- I do get turned on sometimes, but some days it's easy and some days it is so hard, and I never know which it's going to be.
- There is this laundry list of things running through my head and it is impossible to shut it down. I keep trying to get my brain back on task, but it just keeps wandering away.
- Things that used to really turn me on, like books, movies, or watching my partner get undressed, just don't seem to have any impact on me anymore. I could be watching an ad for detergent.
- I feel like such a loser when the women around me talk about being turned on. What does that even mean?

TWO TOTALLY DIFFERENT AROUSAL STORIES

Janet, a forty-two-year-old mother of two teenagers, plunks herself at my table. "My vagina is broken," she says, describing it the way I've heard hundreds of times. "I used to get turned on—a lot! When I would read sexy books or watch sexy movies, I'd get all tingly and excited. And with my husband, he would look at me in a certain way and zing, there went my vagina."

"And now . . . ," I ask.

"Now, NOTHING. All the stuff that he used to do to drive me wild and get me wet, now I find myself having a hard time concentrating. I'm thinking about the stuff I was supposed to do today, I'm thinking about all the stuff I'm supposed to do tomorrow, I just can't stay focused. I don't get turned on. What is wrong with me?"

More than anything, Janet seems angry at herself and confused. She feels like she should be able to will herself into arousal, and that if she just tried harder, she could make it happen.

Emily is a bouncy, twenty-eight-year-old single woman who has no idea what everyone is talking about.

"I can't stand it," she says. "Everyone keeps talking about getting turned on. What the heck does that mean, even? I know something is supposed to be happening to me, but nothing does. I'm not even sure what I'm supposed to feel like. I start dating guys and I want to have sex, but I feel nothing, at least nothing that makes me want to continue. Mostly I feel like it would be more fun if we went to the movies or watched TV or took a long walk." She looks at me, bewildered and lost, and looking way younger than her age. "I feel like a total freak!"

Although the experiences are different, Emily's story is not all that different from Janet's. Neither women is getting aroused. Neither woman is finding that first rung on the ladder.

CAN PROBLEMS WITH AROUSAL GET TREATED?

You know how some days you're just stiff? You can stretch, bend, or take hot showers, but your bones and muscles won't cooperate. Well, what is happening with your body when you're having trouble becoming aroused is similar. Nothing that usually works "fixes" the problem. Please know that there are numerous factors that allow your body to get aroused, many of them out of your short-term control. You can't just turn them off and on at will. Just because you were able to access your arousal yesterday does not mean that you are not trying hard enough today. Beating up on yourself will just make everything worse. You just have to figure out what factors are contributing to the problem. But once you have figured out what might be going on, you can then focus on those solutions that will give you more points in that area.

First of all, let's try to identify whether the problem is "universal" or "situational"; that is, whether you've always got the same problem, or it only happens in one situation. Don't worry; it's not better to have one than the other, it just may mean that your focus may have to be a bit different.

Situational: You do get turned on by some things.
It just feels as though whenever you get started having
sex it is just impossible to keep it going.

You watch sexy movies or read sexy books and feel your body responding, but then somehow, when you climb into bed with your partner, it all seems to fizzle. Now, don't get all upset as you read the description and think, "I can't believe I didn't notice that the hot guy at the gym still turns me on and it's just my husband who leaves me flat! Oh no! It must be my relationship and I guess we're doomed!" That is both not true and not helpful. If you get turned on by a whole host of stimuli, books, movies, billboards, fantasies, but not in other situations where you want to be turned on (say, with your partner), that very well may be good news. It basically means a lot of things are working fine for you (you've got a solid base of points), but you are somehow falling below the threshold you need (100 points) when you are with your partner. You may be interested in Chapters 15–17, which focus on neuroplasticity (learning how to fantasize) and the emotional complications of long-term relationships, or in Chapter 19, about how your kids may be getting in the way of your sex life. The vibrator discussion in Chapter 14 might work well for you as well.

And if you are interested in raising your base threshold through hormones or medications, that can be extremely helpful too. Think about it this way: if your base threshold is a 70, when you are very relaxed (say, at the movies) and seeing things that are very hot to you, that might well add 30 points—which helps you clear the threshold. After a long busy day and tucking two kids into bed, you and your partner whom you love and truly want to have sex with, might only provide 20 points and that bottom rung of the ladder is just not there. Bumping up the base points, by exploring hormonal deficiencies or medications that are making things more difficult, can be very helpful. If you are starting with 80 or 90 points, it makes it much easier to function on a day-to-day basis. So, I wouldn't discount the medical or hormonal route either (Chapters 9–11).

Universal: Absolutely nothing seems to turn you on anymore.

You don't get those "tingles" now. Not when you see the hot fire-fighter who lives down the block and used to get you going. Not when you read or watch erotica. Or if you do get that tingle, it's so few and far between, you almost can't remember the last time. Books, movies, or discussions that used to get you thinking about sex, or that everyone else seemed to respond to, seem to do nothing erotic for you. Or nothing "sexy" ever did seem to turn you on—you theoretically want to have sex, but nothing happens in your body. It never did, and you are pretty hopeless that it ever will.

If nothing turns you on anymore, I'm going to go out on a limb here and say that it sounds like something significant has shifted physiologically (or chemically) for you. If your arousal seems to have died on the vine, take a good look at Chapter 10. You'll need the help of a physician who is supportive of the use of hormones for sexual problems and is trained in that area.

You also should have a physician review any medications you are taking, because some very commonly used drugs are arousal killers. If drugs are affecting your ability to become aroused, it will be very, very difficult to make up the missing points in other areas. You really need those points! (Chapter 11 addresses some of the most common culprits.)

While medical components may be undergirding the issue, you may be suffering from a secondary effect: your brain is out of practice and isn't working the way it once did. Studies on the new field of neuroplasticity have made it far clearer how much your fantasy life can develop or stagnate depending on whether it's been used or not. There's a whole chapter on that as well (Chapter 16). In this case, you really do need to focus on your brain for these changes. But that doesn't mean you can just will your head back into the game. It will take some time and focus and work to get that part of your brain functioning the way you want it to. Vibrators, because they provide so much stimulation, can also be incredibly helpful (Chapter 14).

If you feel like you really and truly have never been aroused, get thee to a sex therapist. This is a hard road to walk alone. There are drugs you can use that can make this road easier (Chapters 9 and 11), there are exercises that you can do to get your erotic brain to function (Chapter 16) and toys that you can use that might jump-start your brain (Chapter 14), but when you don't have a past template to work from, you may need a bit of outside help. You want a therapist who respects that our sexual response is partly in our head and partly in our body, someone who can help you sort out the points so that you can reclaim them for yourself. Here's what you don't want: a therapist who is going to blame your lack of ability to become aroused on past trauma that you don't remember or past activities that don't seem particularly relevant. Although exploring your history can be helpful and working through past traumas is a necessary starting point, you want a therapist who can join you in your goal to find solutions that work for you and helps you fix the problems. You may want to take this book with you to your appointment with your sex therapist and explore together the ways in which you think you can gather points. Check Appendix II (page 271) for help in finding a sex therapist.

What if it actually is the relationship?

If you DO get turned on in many situations but never when you are with your partner, then you need to figure out whether something specific is going on in the relationship that is causing you to turn off. Relationships are complicated, and everyone has moments in time when they wonder why they even partnered with the person they are with; there will be times that you might feel that way for a few weeks. If that's you, and you find that you love your partner and are theoretically interested in sex with them, but just seem to have trouble finding that spark, then focus on the solutions I list at the end of this chapter.

But it's important to realize that a few weeks of feeling, "Why is my partner such a mess? John from work is always pulled together and charming" is not the same thing as feeling as though you are with someone who actively turns you off—all the time. And you can't remember the last time you, even theoretically, wanted to have sex with this person. If this is the case, it might be a good idea to find a marriage counselor—but only one who is comfortable talking about sex AND communication.

Many couples counselors are comfortable with the communication part of a relationship and are much less comfortable with the practical part of the sex life of a couple. Some are even convinced that if you fix the communication issues in the relationship, the sex will follow. That has not been my experience. Couples often have to actively work at their sex life, even when the relationship is humming along quite well. Many people are in perfectly lovely and functional relationships, but sex is still a problem. So, if your relationship is having problems and you are going to a couples counselor to address the relationship first, I would still encourage you to find a couples counselor who can not only work with you to help you navigate or repair your relationship, but also actively work with you on your sex life and understand why sex is such an issue. So, you will need to see a therapist who is truly comfortable with addressing specific sexual issues and competent at giving you specific suggestions to fix things. I've included a guide to finding a therapist (see Appendix II, page 271). Sex is your presenting problem and you want a counselor who will bring it up, discuss it with you, and keep it on the table.

It may help you clarify by checking out Chapter 15, on limerence. But remember, there is a world of difference between couples who are not thrillingly attracted to each other, bored, or unmoved by their partner, and those couples where a partner actively feels turned off, disgusted, or too angry to consider sex.

No matter who you are, getting turned on, finding yourself aroused when you are having sex, be it by yourself or with a partner, is critically important to having a great sex life. Identifying the parameters of the problem is the first step in trying to fix it. And you need to believe me that it truly is fixable.

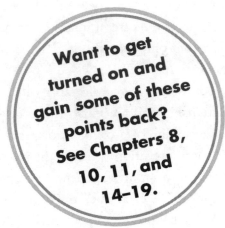

Want to get turned on and gain some of these points back? See Chapters 8, 10, 11, and 14–19.

CHAPTER 6

ORGASM

It's Not All "When Harry Met Sally"

> − 30 to 60 points
>
> *Your lack of orgasm makes sex less . . . fun, or is really making you frustrated.*
>
> *Your lack of orgasm may also significantly affect your arousal and desire.*

We've all seen the sex scenes. Clothes seem to fall off by themselves. (No struggling with bras or hoodies?) The penis magically finds its way into the vagina in two seconds flat, without a hand guiding it in. (Penises are not actually homing pigeons). The woman writhes, screams, and moans. Her orgasm is explosive, and she's loud. It always happens the first time, and it's *exactly* at the same time as her partner. Least realistic of all? There's never a wet spot—or a fight about who has to sleep on it.

Sorry, folks. That kind of orgasm is about as realistic as growing your hair long enough to let someone climb up and rescue you in your tower. And the problem is, it's the only story many of us have heard. Movies have probably created more misconceptions about sex than parents have. (Which, frankly, is saying something.) But many women have not had orgasms, and it's not automatic—it's something you can learn. Bottom line: if you have never experienced orgasm, you are not alone.

When I say "never" had an orgasm, I mean it in any way, including masturbation, manual or oral stimulation, vibrator, or intercourse. Sex is about much more than orgasm, and there are people with a satisfying sex life who do not experience orgasm. But for many, it can be physically and emotionally frustrating not to have one. Most women (hovering somewhere around 94 percent) can have orgasms.[1] There is a direct correlation between ability to experience orgasm and sexual satisfaction (as most women who have them will generally assure you). The opposite, that the inability to achieve orgasm lowers a woman's level of sexual satisfaction, is also often true. Orgasms are good for you. They bring blood into the vaginal area, keeping your vagina moist and supple, and they are relaxing.[2] Best of all, they (usually) feel great.

For some women, it's harder than others. Some women need high levels of stimulation, whereas others do not; some need chemical or technical help; some 5 percent may never have an orgasm at all.[3] It's a combination of learning about your body, your brain, relaxation, and finding what kind of stimulation works for you—most people, women and men, first learn to experience orgasm through masturbation. It takes time and patience. Your mind and body are in this together. (By the way, if someone says they guarantee you an orgasm, that's either just bunk, or their definition of an orgasm isn't in the dictionary.)

WHAT IS AN ORGASM?

An orgasm begins with what we call the "excitement phase." Typically, as a woman becomes turned on, her breasts swell, her nipples become erect, and her uterus tips downward. At this point, more stimulation of her clitoris, vulva, and vagina will bring on general body tension, and increase blood flow to the vulvar/vaginal area. As the blood keeps building in the vulvar/vaginal area, a woman will experience her genitals as tense and tight. This feeling, which usually also involves feelings of tingling, swelling, and wetness, is generally experienced as pleasurable.

Once the stimulation reaches a crescendo, the nerve endings, which are overloaded with stimulation, "shoot off" to release the neurological tension, and then a series of involuntary contractions occur in response. The contractions, which are happening in the uterus and vagina, carry the blood away from the genitals and back to the rest of the body (unless the woman tries to have another orgasm). As the orgasm resolves, most women find the tension fades away and they feel relaxed, both in their genitals and often the rest of their body.

WHAT DO ORGASM PROBLEMS LOOK LIKE?

Here's how women generally describe their difficulty with having orgasms:

- Um . . . What's an orgasm?
- I can have an orgasm by myself, but never with a partner.
- I can have an orgasm with a partner, but not from vaginal intercourse.
- I have orgasms in a totally weird way.
- I used to orgasm fine, but these days, orgasms take so much darn work!
- My orgasms used to be good . . . now they barely register on the Richter scale.

THE THREE SIDES OF AN ORGASM

When a woman tells me that she has trouble having an orgasm, I look at three factors: what is happening in her genitals, what is happening in her brain, and what is her hormone profile. These are the questions I ask:

- Are you getting enough genital stimulation to bring on an orgasm?
- Are you getting enough mental stimulation to allow for the orgasm?

- Are your hormones and blood flow aligned with the ability to have an orgasm?

Genital Stimulation

Each woman needs a particular type of genital stimulation to activate the nerve endings and experience the chain reaction that is an orgasm. Women prefer and react differently to different stimulation. Some women can orgasm just by squeezing their legs together. Others need a strong vibrator to provide sufficient stimulation. It is all very individual, and the only real way to ascertain what you need is by trial and error.

Mental Stimulation

To orgasm, a woman needs the parts of the brain that connect to her nerve endings to be stimulated as well. We're understanding more about neuroplasticity, the study of how thinking can actually change your brain. Often, women who are having trouble with orgasm are the same women who say they don't fantasize, or don't get turned on by their thoughts. Learning to use your erotic brain is a challenging yet incredibly rewarding project. And this may be the place where you can get additional points.

Hormones and Blood Flow

Blood flow is important for orgasmic functioning. Some new research shows that insufficient blood flow to the vaginal area can prevent the clitoris from becoming properly engorged and impedes orgasm. Some preliminary studies have shown that women, immediately after exercising, have increased blood flow, increased lubrication, become aroused more quickly, and orgasm more easily.[4]

As you get older, you may see differences in your blood circulation, or nerve or brain functioning. If the blood flow in the vagina is insufficient, it will not fully engorge the clitoris—much like a man who can't get an erection. If your clitoris does not become engorged, you may not have the intensity of orgasm that you are used to. This can also sometimes be caused by certain medical conditions, medications, or surgeries.[5] The medications you may be taking can also be affecting your ability to experience orgasm, particularly if you are taking antidepressants. Additionally, birth control pills can throw off the balance of hormones and create an inability to orgasm. Neurotransmitters in the brain may not be working as efficiently as they used to.

Hormones are also a critical component of normal sexual response. Low levels of testosterone-related hormones that are often associated with perimenopausal and postmenopausal women can have a large impact on both a woman's level of desire and her level of response. Understanding the hormone balance is a new area for most physicians, and most don't know that, if you have experienced pleasurable orgasm in the past, it is likely that with the proper combination of medical and emotional support, you can do so again.

"JUST DEAL WITH IT": CHERYL'S STORY

Cheryl is a smart, no-nonsense fifty-two-year-old decked out in a business suit and wire-frame glasses. She seems rather uncomfortable being in the position of asking for help.

"I think I'm different than most of the other women you see here," she starts out. "And I don't really think you can help me."

As she continues, I wish I could make this easier for her. "When my husband and I had sex," she explains, "I'd always orgasm, sometimes more than once. I had orgasms from his hand, from his mouth, from his penis. But five years ago, they started to get harder to have. I'd have to concentrate, which I never had to do before. And then, to make matters worse, it took forever. I started feeling guilty making him work so hard."

Here she smiles at me for the first time. "I mean, how fair is it to make a guy go down on you for twenty minutes?"

"But the truth is," she says, "he's great about it, and I could have lived with that. But now the orgasms barely register on the radar. They are these little ripples. I start to feel like it is just not worth it. It's so frustrating! You know, if I had never had them before maybe I wouldn't care so much." (Sorry Cheryl, I beg to differ.) "But it feels like sex is frustrating and unfulfilling and I just don't want to do it anymore. My husband is pretty sad. So am I."

"And why don't you think we can help?" I ask.

"Well, I spoke to my gynecologist and she said"—I grit my teeth, because I know what's coming—"It's just a part of getting older. Deal with it.'"

This story is so common I see it playing out again and again in my office. Discounting the hormonal or other physiological changes in older women just leaves them in an untenable situation.

In Cheryl's case, physical factors seemed to be at play. We put her on bupropion, a medication that raises the dopamine (a.k.a. pleasure hormone), and within a month, Cheryl was having her old orgasms again.

Bottom line, Cheryl did not just have to "deal with it." And neither do you.

Now let me break down specific and common orgasm issues that come up. These might save you months or years of insecurity or heartache. And hopefully they will lead you closer to regaining your points.

"I CAN'T HAVE AN ORGASM THROUGH INTERCOURSE."

Contrary to popular myth, most women don't achieve orgasm through intercourse alone. Only 30 percent of them do![6] That is 3 in 10 women. And if you don't trust me, know that the real expert, *Cosmopolitan* magazine, prints that information at least once a month. And if you don't trust *Cosmo*, large-scale scientific studies say the same thing: For the majority of women, the position and the way in which the clitoris is being stimulated through intercourse is not conducive to orgasm—meaning, there's no way intercourse alone can produce an orgasm. For some women, orgasming through intercourse is the equivalent of bringing a man to orgasm by rubbing his testicles. It is unlikely that without proper stimulation of the penis, he will reach orgasm. It's unlikely that without proper stimulation of your clitoris, you will reach orgasm.

When you can't orgasm through intercourse, you are not anorgasmic—merely typical! But you may have to spend some time mourning your fantasy that penile penetration will bring an orgasm and the best sex of your life.

Luckily, there are so many good alternatives. Your partner can stimulate you manually either during, prior to, or after intercourse; you can stimulate yourself manually during intercourse; or you can try out a vibrator. There are even vibrators that are meant specifically to use while you are having intercourse (although frankly, I'm still holding out for a better model, because in our experience none of them work very well).

"I ORGASM IN A WEIRD WAY."

Here's a story that repeats itself often in my office. I'm sitting with a new patient. She is usually some version of polished, bright, successful, and articulate. She informs me that she can never have orgasms with her partner in the room, and I proceed to ask the obvious follow-up:

"Can you tell me a little about how you usually have orgasm on your own?"

She avoids my eyes. She looks at the floor. She looks out the window. She hems and haws. She looks just above my head. I decide I should just put her out of her misery.

"Do you have them on your stomach, rubbing against something—the floor, a blanket, a stuffed animal . . . ?" My voice trails off as her jaw drops. She looks at me as though I have just spontaneously combusted.

"HOW DID YOU KNOW THAT???"

As far as I can tell, there are two potential answers to that question:

1. I am a brilliant mind reader and know what my patients are going to say before they say it, *or*
2. It's actually pretty common.

Patients struggle to tell me the "weird way" they orgasm all the time. Most of the women who orgasm easiest lying on their stomach and rubbing something, think they are the *only* women in the world who do so. Sometimes it takes forty-five minutes (and up to two weeks) for them to tell me the deep dark secret. Since I estimate about one-quarter of all women masturbate on their stomach, that's a lot of women who think they're sexual deviants.

And why is it that every single woman who has an orgasm on her stomach thinks she's some aberration? Maybe, just maybe, it's because *every single damn movie has the heroine orgasm on her back*? Even those movies that show women masturbating—and they're few and far between—show them moaning and groaning usually in the missionary position. I'm not a director, but my theory is it makes for better footage. That means most women have no idea what positions women orgasm in all the time. And if you have a very limited idea of what normal is, you get thrown by reality.

When women are forced to define themselves as abnormal or aberrant when what they're doing is incredibly common, it does real damage to their self-esteem. And this is too bad, because learning to have an orgasm on your stomach makes perfect sense. A little girl in bed starts touching herself and rolls inadvertently onto her bunched-up blanket, her pillow, or favorite teddy bear. Wow. That feels good. Next time, she tries it on purpose. Voilà: the road to a perfect orgasm.

I had a patient once who was an avid hiker. She could only orgasm while rubbing up against a climbing rope or pole. I have met any number of women who have had their first orgasm climbing on a rope in gym class, so I wasn't particularly thrown. But by the time she told me, she sounded like she was confessing to murder. She was so embarrassed she had never told her husband of twenty years or her therapist of six years. We began to think through ways we could re-create a climbing rope in her bedroom, and, eventually, how to tell her husband. She didn't go with my suggestion to have a pole installed and incorporate pole-dancing into her sex life, but it gave her a good laugh. Once she felt free enough to tell her husband, just the weight of revealing her secret opened her up to better sex, and they ultimately incorporated orgasms into their sex life.

"HOW DO I TRANSLATE MY WEIRD WAY OF ORGASMING INTO SEX WITH MY PARTNER?"

Here's a question I feel doesn't deserve a smart-ass answer. Although there is no right or wrong way to orgasm, some ways are easier to share with a partner. While squeezing your legs together or climbing a rope are fine and reasonable ways to orgasm, they do pose significant challenges once you put another person in the equation. Orgasms on a rope with two folks are harder. But listen: you just learned how to ride a unicycle, and now you want to ride a bicycle. You are not kinky, or aberrant! So, here are some suggestions to deal with the situation.

Tell your partner. It is hard to make changes in a relationship if you don't explain the situation. To do this, you need to accept that there is nothing inherently wrong with you and you are totally normal and not kinky or crazy (see above). So, come clean. And if you have been faking orgasm until now, please stop. Instead, show your partner how it's done. If they see how you do it, the two of you can work together to come up with a solution. Try not to be embarrassed. They will probably think watching you orgasm is a total turn-on.

Build your orgasms as you currently have them into your sex life. Can you rub up against his leg, his penis, his hand? Can you rub up against another object while he comes inside you from behind? Or after intercourse, roll over and have him touch you while you make yourself orgasm?

If you want to try to "retrain your orgasms," make sure you do it gradually, baby step by baby step and with a strong sense of humor. So, you want to learn to orgasm on your back? Use your favorite rub-against object, get yourself close, and then roll over still using it. If it doesn't work, try another variation. Just don't ever get angry at yourself or feel as though your entire sex life depends on it, because it doesn't.

Try a strong vibrator. A higher level of stimulation may make the difference, so now might be the time to consider a vibrator (Chapter 14). You may be able to orgasm on your back with a vibrator—but then, no complaining "I can only orgasm with a vibrator," please! When you are trying to change the way you have an orgasm, making the orgasm easier to achieve is important.

"ORGASMS TAKE SO MUCH WORK . . . AND THERE IS SO LITTLE PAYOFF!"

This is one of the most common complaints I hear. It's often from older women who find it is significantly more difficult to orgasm, and that the orgasms themselves are getting weaker and wimpy. I also hear it from women who have recently gone through childbirth. When well-meaning counselors or physicians tell women that they should just live with weaker and weaker orgasms they are (rightly) furious. *I KNOW how to have an orgasm*, they think. *I had them for the first 15 years of my adult life. And I KNOW what an orgasm feels like, and this is NOT IT.*

The truth is, I love these patients, because these are easy problems to resolve: If you know how to have an orgasm, you can almost always get them back. It may take making friends with vibrators (Chapter 14) because you may now need a higher, stronger level of stimulation than you used to. It may mean trying hormone therapy (Chapter 10), or medications to rebuild your neurotransmitter dopamine (Chapter 11), or getting PRP (platelet-rich plasma) injections (Chapter 11). It may need a combination of those things. Sometimes, you need to retrain your brain to access the really hot, sexy fantasies (Chapter 16).

I will tell you what I responded to Regina, who sat in my office crying "I thought for sure you would tell me that this was just the way life is after fifty-five and I should just get used to it." "Nope, Regina. Please don't get used to it. Let's get you back your old orgasms." And we did!

"I'VE NEVER HAD AN ORGASM."

Just because you have never experienced an orgasm doesn't mean that you can't. I'm assuming if you're reading this book, you've tried to have an orgasm but haven't succeeded. That can be incredibly frustrating.

In my experience, women who have never had an orgasm usually fall in one of three categories:

1. The first category are those women who actually aren't really getting very turned on at all. They are left cold by any sexual activity and never get into throwing range of having an orgasm. Often, these women indicate their lack of arousal by saying "I don't have an orgasm," but it's more likely they have an arousal problem than an orgasm problem. Those in that category need to start working on their arousal before they get hung up on having an orgasm.

   But if you are in that category, please realize that you have to learn to walk before you can run. Quadrant II, Arousal

(Chapter 5) describes that problem. In that case you need to consider those factors that could be giving you more points. You can do that by training or accessing your erotic mind (Chapters 15 and 16), learning to use the right vibrator (Chapter 14), or taking hormones and modifying medication (Chapters 8–10). Once you start getting aroused, then you can start focusing on having an orgasm—if it doesn't happen by itself!

2. Another category is made up of women who get incredibly turned on, feel they are just about to have an orgasm, and then it fizzles. They wear out their hands, their partner's mouth, or the batteries on their vibrator, but they just can't cross the finish line. It's incredibly irritating and physically frustrating.

   Unfortunately, solving this problem can be difficult, because we don't understand enough about the neurological level you need to set off an orgasm. We've learned something from the fact that women who go on antianxiety medications that work on the serotonin receptors experience the same thing:[7] it gives us a clue that a too-high serotonin level may be the culprit. But it doesn't tell us how to solve the problem.

   If this is you, the first thing you need to know is that you are not crazy, and you are not doing anything wrong. In fact, part of the difficulty is that you're doing everything right, and it's not working. You can try to garner points by switching up the lineup: using a stronger vibrator (Chapter 14), or different fantasies (Chapter 16). Some very smart neuropsychologists as well as BDSM practitioners have suggested that adding in some additional nerve stimulation, such as minor pain (twisted nipples, a slap), can help women get over that threshold. However, there is no data to support this theory, and very little anecdotal evidence to support it. Using a platelet-rich blood treatment to engage the clitoris is also worth a try (Chapter 11).

3. Then, there are women who can get incredibly turned on, and somehow, they know when they are finished, even if they don't

feel the explosion (large or small) in the way other women do. These women seem to be having an orgasm, even if they are not actually feeling it. Sometimes, they feel reasonably okay, since their body does return to a relaxed state, and they don't feel the frustration of not orgasming. However, they do feel that everyone else is having a better time than they are. They are supposed to feel their orgasms and they don't feel like their experience mirrors the screaming you find in the movies. These are what we, in our center, call "subclinical" orgasm. If you have these, you have a few choices. You can decide that your orgasms are adequate and that you don't want to waste your time chasing a rainbow. Or you can feel that although you are fine as you are, it would be nice to experiment with switching up your method of orgasming. If you do, be sure to start slowly and keep expectations open: PRP shots (Chapter 11), stronger or different vibrators (Chapter 14), internal and external stimulation, anal stimulation, or hotter or different fantasies (Chapter 16) may produce a different kind of orgasm.

But one note of caution: I always remember the O. Henry story about the exceptionally beautiful woman with a beauty mark. Her husband was obsessed with it: he wanted her face to be perfect and couldn't get past it. But in the attempt to remove it, they destroyed her face—and her beauty! I am assuming you get my analogy. If you are trying to have an orgasm that you feel more, that's great. Just don't destroy your entire sex life in the process.

"WHAT IF IT REALLY IS ALL IN MY HEAD?"

There *are* women who get "blocked" psychologically from experiencing orgasm. Typically, those are the ones who can reach orgasm through masturbation, but can't when there's a partner in the room, or they have suffered a recent trauma that impeded their regular sex life.

Where I differ from many other sex therapists is that I disagree with the idea that problems in a relationship, untreated abuse from decades ago, or simple unhappiness can rear its head at age 35, or 55, or 75, and stop you from having orgasms in any context. That just hasn't been my experience with patients, and, as a clinician, I think intentionally or not the therapist is simply blaming the patient, or is uncomfortable admitting that they don't know or can't help. Either way, I just don't buy it. And neither should you.

Please be sure your doctor or therapist doesn't assume your problem is emotional. If you're having trouble with an orgasm because of a physical problem, or you simply need better techniques, all the talk therapy in the world won't make any difference. If you've read this far, you know that low hormone levels, medical conditions, and medications, such as birth control pills, antianxiety drugs, or antidepressants, can all contribute to a woman's inability to experience an orgasm. You also get that learning to use the erotic part of your brain, becoming comfortable in your body, and having your brain and genitals communicate with each other are key.

If you have experienced trauma or are truly having emotional or psychological issues, such as shame or anxiety, you should still use a general therapist who is comfortable talking about sex and working to improve your sex life. Bottom line: it's never all in your head.

Want some of these points back? See Chapters 8–11, 14, 16, 17, and 19.

CHAPTER 7

DESIRE

"I'd Rather Be Doing the Laundry"

> −45 to 80 points
>
> *You may have lost some, or all, of your 45 desire points.*
>
> *Your low desire may also result in lost points from arousal and orgasm.*

"I love my partner, but I don't desire him anymore."

"It's just not worth the effort."

"I can't drag myself to do it."

Desire is one of our most complex and mysterious feelings. It's a mix of hormones, chemicals, relationships, and self-awareness. It's eroticism, passion, simple physical need, and love. Although desire is not the be-all and end-all of good sex, it's often central. And there are millions of women who are afraid there is something very wrong with them because they don't feel enough desire to want to have sex with their partner.

Low libido, which we commonly call low desire, affects both your relationship and your sense of self. Often, women with low libido don't feel as happy, or as vibrant, as they did when they felt it was functioning well. They once had a libido and liked it. Their libido is inherent to who they are, not simply a factor in a relationship, and they miss the feeling of being alive that sexual desire gave them.

When you *are* in a relationship and desire isn't there, it can seem like a chasm that can't be breached. Lack of desire can have significant ramifications on a partner's feeling about you, and about themselves and their own desirability. It can significantly affect your own feelings

83

about your role in the relationship. As one woman put it, "Frankly, I couldn't care less if I never had sex again. But my marriage is paying a real price, and I can't imagine us making it as a couple unless I fix this problem."

Low desire means that you don't want to have sex. It doesn't mean that you can't get turned on, or have good sex (that would be an arousal problem, and it's a separate quadrant). It means that "wanting" is gone or ridiculously faded. And it makes it very hard to enter into or continue a sexual relationship. It's like eating when you are not at all hungry.

It also doesn't only happen to those of us over fifty. Women in their forties, thirties, and twenties experience low desire—and some women feel they've never experienced desire at all. It can exist alongside other problems, like pain, or the inability to have an orgasm, or an inability to become aroused. But it can also exist alone. You can have low desire, but still enjoy sex once you're doing it.

Libido is complicated, because it gets wrapped up in so many other problems. Take pain. If you feel it's going to hurt every time you have sex, how could you maintain desire? Avoiding intercourse because of pain can sometimes mean just that. But women with high desire who have severe pain with intercourse will find other ways to have sex. They will have oral sex or manual sex (using their hands) or some other kind of sex that feels great, leads to orgasm, but doesn't involve penetration.

Women often mix up problems with arousal and desire. They think if their body doesn't respond, get turned on, if they are having trouble quieting that to-do list in their head (which are all symptoms of arousal problems), then they must have a desire problem. But these are separate—if often related—problems. Yes, when your arousal and orgasms are humming along, that can help you want sex more, which can have a positive effect on desire. But there are definitely women who have great arousal and orgasm—their body responds quickly and well—and when they get started having sex, the sex is fun and feels great, and even then, they *still* don't want to do it again.

Although it seems counterintuitive, a woman who can respond easily and have good orgasms can still not want sex. A quick way to see whether your problem is probably one of a lack of desire or a lack of arousal is this: If I waved a magic wand over you and you knew that you could get aroused and orgasm easily, would you be happy? Would you want to have more sex? If your response is "YES. YES!" then that tells me that we are probably looking at a problem of arousal. That is not generally the response of low-desire women. In those cases, women may look at me sadly and say, "But I do get turned on. The sex can be pretty good. I just don't seem to have any interest in doing it again."

We live in a busy world and many of us lead complicated lives. Some of the craziness of life can be controlled and some of it can't. That means most of us will experience low libido at some point, caused by external conditions: we have stress and anxiety, less-than-perfect relationships, and not enough time to relax and regroup. This alone can wreak havoc on a woman's libido. Emily Nagoski discusses this powerfully in her book *Come As You Are*, in which she describes the "brakes" in our sexual psyche that inhibit us from being able to respond easily to sexual cues.[1]

But there are external reasons a woman suffers from a low libido, ones that can't be fixed by stress levels or time off. Your libido is affected by physiological conditions in your body: hormone levels, vitamin deficiencies, and neurotransmitter health. Low libido can be a symptom of depression. It can hint at thyroid problems or anemia. It can be caused by permanent conditions in a relationship: lack of intimacy, lack of trust, lack of time. It can be caused by personal struggles of our own: a dislike of our body, a general unhappiness with our life, a lack of time or energy.[2]

Michelle, a forty-five-year-old attorney, is happily married for eighteen years with three kids. "Whenever I have sex with my husband," Michelle says, "I get turned on, it feels great, and I have an orgasm. But then it's a week later and I'm counting the days since we've had sex, wondering when I 'have' to do it again."

Low libido can also look like Marjorie, a thirty-six-year-old stay-at-home mom of two. Nine years ago, when she was suffering from anxiety attacks, she went on a number of medications. "I went from being this girl who wanted sex a lot—and I mean a lot—to suddenly being uninterested. I used to masturbate all the time, and I always had a boyfriend. And suddenly, nothing.

"Then, I met and married my husband, and things are the same. He deserves to have a wife who wants him, who desires him. And you know what? I remember the me who wanted sex. I really liked her. I deserve to get her back!"

Yes, Marjorie—you do.

That doesn't mean if you don't want to have sex every day, you have low libido. Everyone has their own threshold for how much sex they want, need, and can fit into their life. That changes over our lifetime, depending on schedule, partner, children, and many other factors. Low desire can be natural, and a healthy libido can weather the normal ups and downs of a crazy life and bounce back after a relatively short shutdown.

Only you can tell whether your current desire for sex doesn't fit into the life you want and have planned for yourself. Only you can tell whether you *desire* to feel more desire. In a way, it's simple: you need to decide if you have low libido. And if you do, and if it's making you unhappy, you should take it seriously—and understand it can be fixed.

WHAT LOW LIBIDO LOOKS LIKE

Here are the many ways women often describe their feelings of low desire:

- "I used to love sex. What's happened to me?"
- "I feel confused and ashamed that I can't seem to want something I want to want."

- "I don't miss it, but if I don't do something about it, my relationship is going to fall apart."
- "Date? Why bother?"
- "I feel like I'm cheating my partner from the best part of me."
- "I love them so much, and yet I dread, absolutely dread, the idea of having sex with them!"

Your lack of sex drive changes your sense of self.

Time after time, women say to me that they miss having their libido because their sexual desire made them feel younger, more alive, and connected to the world around them. Those who used to have a strong libido often feel the loss of something special and important to them. They feel it in their lack of interest with masturbation, not noticing attractive people around them and, if they are not in a relationship, even in their lack of interest in dating and meeting new people.

You feel like you are living in an alternate universe.

Women who have never been able to access their sexual desire often say they feel crazy or weird when their friends talk about sex and they don't know what the fuss is about. Some of them say they feel like the world is using a language they just don't understand. They worry they will never feel "normal."

Your lack of sex drive is hurting your relationship.

Some experts feel that if the woman personally isn't bothered by her lack of desire, if she is merely motivated by her relationship, then there is no real problem to fix. They believe that low desire is just a modern construct created by our society, that pressure being placed on her from our current culture or her intimate partner (or other sources) is not a valid reason to look for help.

I don't agree with that perspective. You can be okay with your lack of desire and still feel it is having a detrimental impact on your relationship. For some women, this is the motivation to fix the problem.

Working on your libido to help your relationship and/or your partner seems as real and positive to me as working on your communication style to help your relationship or your partner. Romantic relationships and partnering are powerful commitments, and often critical to who we are and the life we want to live. Working on those areas that will keep those relationships healthy and happy is important and meaningful. And often, romantic relationships will not remain intact and joyful when the sex life isn't there.

THE FOUR LEVELS OF DESIRE

Over the years I've developed a ranking system to help women assess their own level of desire on a continuum. It goes from 1 to 4, with 1 having the most desire and 4 having the least. Think of it as a snapshot, and a starting point to assessing your current level of desire.

1. Sex is one of your favorite hobbies.

No one ever needs to remind you that you haven't had sex in a week. As a matter of fact, you often spontaneously think about sex, feel sexual, initiate sex with your partner (if you have one), or masturbate regularly if you don't. You start thinking about it on your own and you'll generally do something about it. You're happy to discuss sex with the people around you when it comes up because sex is a fun, important part of your life.

There are, indeed, some women in this category, but not, by my experience, a whole hell of a lot. This group tends to encompass young women and a small select few who seem to be graced with an innately high libido. This is a great space to be in, but perhaps not entirely necessary for a good, fun, spontaneous sex life.

2. You say, "Sure, honey, I'll be there in a minute," and mean it.

You may not be spontaneously thinking of sex that often, but you are happy to oblige when your partner initiates. Or the spirit may move you to masturbate when you see something that turns you on. Or, if you decide that you miss having had sex for a while or feel that it would be good to have an orgasm (to relax, to feel good, to fall asleep), it's just not a big deal to get in the mood. Usually, if you start doing the things that turn you on (kissing or touching your partner, fantasizing, or looking at something sexy), you find yourself wanting sex.

This model was first described by a gynecologist, Rosemary Basson, in 2000[3] when she suggested that this, for most women, better described their experience than the classic Masters and Johnson response cycle,[4] which purported that spontaneous desire always kicked in first, before arousal and orgasm. But, honestly, that's not how many women function. Many women get started having sexual thoughts or experiences, kissing, touching, fantasizing, because they want to "want" to have sex. This model is a better description of many women's experience, and most women who exist in this plane of desire are happy with their sex life.

3. Sex? How about a good game of cards?

You know you should want sex, but somehow the idea of actually doing it is overwhelming. You avoid it, perhaps by spending twenty minutes in the shower, hoping he'll fall asleep before you get to bed. You are probably having sex on some kind of regular basis, whether weekly, monthly, or bi-yearly, and you think with dread about when you'll have to have sex again and try to put it off for as many days as you can. When you do finally have sex, you try hard, since you love your partner. If you are not partnered, you probably haven't fantasized, thought about sex, or masturbated in months or years. This may be affecting your interest in dating altogether. You may also feel sad because it wasn't always this way.

4. You'd rather have your toenails removed with no anesthesia.

You really, really want to want to have sex. But the thought, frankly, makes you want to cower. It's making you panicked. It's also destroying the relationship, or your partner's sense of self-esteem, or your view of yourself. If you are partnered, you might be having sex once a month (or for some of you brave souls, once a week), but you don't know how much longer it will continue because it is becoming unbearable. You might even wish your partner would have an affair to relieve some of his/her tension, or that your partner gives you an ultimatum. And if you are alone? Well, you are perfectly happy to stay alone.

Usually, when a woman ranks at a level 3 or 4 in low desire, we see cracks develop in the relationship. Either one or both of the couple is often angry. Little things that her partner does that might otherwise be shrugged off, start to really irritate her, and her partner feels rejected. They often both feel sad. Often, couples in this situation barely touch anymore. Why? Well, the woman (legitimately) feels that if she kisses her partner, cuddles up against them at night, or snuggles on the sofa, they will take that as a signal to initiate a sexual encounter. To avoid yet another painful rejection, she avoids any type of contact at all. But this functions as a double whammy on the partner. "Not only are we never having sex," they'll say, "but we don't even hold hands or kiss anymore." It's a loss of intimacy as well as sexuality. This is one of the most classic—and heartbreaking— secondary developments of low libido. And it's a terrible stalemate. Everyone is right.

Women often describe a general tension, irritability, or snappishness in their partner. "He's always in such a grumpy mood these days," one woman says. Another confesses, "He gets angry at me or the kids so easily." And she's not imagining things. If connection is tied up with physical intimacy—as it often is for men—a partner will feel alone, unloved, and unconnected, physically as well as emotionally. Women often have many ways to be physically intimate: they have woman friends with whom they are emotionally close, they hug and touch friends and their children. People who need to have sex find that the lack of sexual contact is almost unbearable.

This can lead to high levels of tension and stress in relationships that may feel totally unrelated to the sexual issues.

LOW DESIRE CAN BE TREATED

Maybe you've tried those easy remedies like "schedule some time together," "buy some sexy lingerie," and "try it in the bathtub." Either nothing is working or even the idea of trying those things makes you want to burst into tears of frustration. Now what?

Treating low desire involves first figuring out what combination of factors has created the situation. Could a personal struggle be affecting your libido? Is it event-specific? Has your partner changed, or the circumstances of your life changed?

The critical piece is to figure out what's missing and then, what can be changed. Some things are fixable, and unfortunately, some things are just not. Once you figure out what elements are causing your low desire, you can decide what to work on alone, with a partner, or by going to a professional.

Here are the questions that you need to answer, and they function essentially as a decision tree.

"Is my low desire relationship-specific?"

You're fantasizing about your personal trainer, having dreams about old boyfriends, and masturbate a few times a week. But all those feelings seem to melt into thin air with your partner. In fact, not only is your partner not adding points, he's actually taking some away.

You need to answer this question: Do you not want to have sex, or do you just not want to have sex with your partner? If you still fantasize, masturbate, or have sexual dreams, but you are ranking as a 4 with your partner, low desire may not really be your problem. This is a case where talk therapy either alone or couples therapy can be extraordinarily useful. If your partner doesn't want to go with you, you might want to start out alone.

You want a counselor who will bring it up, discuss it with you, put it on the table, and make specific suggestions. I'll say it again: sex is your presenting problem, so make sure that you find a counselor who is really and truly comfortable dealing with sex. Chapters 15–18 may be helpful here.

"I don't think it's my partner. I think it's me."

You don't really fantasize or think about sex much at all, and when you do, it's because you are reading or watching something sexy, not looking at your partner naked. But when you haven't seen them in a while or you're on vacation, you're happy to have sex. This is good news: all that might mean is that you are hovering around or just below your 100-point threshold, and your partner is not providing those extra points. Now, you just have to figure out where you can get your additional points from: hormones, shifts in the relationship, shifts in your lifestyle, possibly medications (Chapters 10, 11, and 15–18).

"Is my low desire environmental?"

Lack of sleep, stress, too much clutter, too many things constantly running around your brain: all of these things can take away points. Unfortunately, sometimes you can't do much about them. But there may be serious ways to restructure your life to create some space for extra points. When Samantha came to see me, she described her crazy life: She was in medical school, had a young child, and had a husband who was feeling despondent because his wife never wanted to have sex with him. It took some work and some talk to unravel some of the crazy expectations she put on herself. Did she really need a perfectly put-together home and to cook everything organic from scratch? She needed (and I mean, needed) more than the five hours of sleep she was getting. Our work focused on finding some space in her over-whelming life, where she could take a hot bath twice a month and decompress, or getting just a small bit of more childcare that would allow her to sleep a few more hours a week. Having more adequate sleep and even just a small window to stop, breathe, fantasize, and focus on her own body, ultimately turned things around. Sometimes, we have more control over our environment than we think. Take a look at Chapters 15, 16, and 19 (even if you don't have kids, 19 might be helpful). See what changes seem practical and doable. If many environmental changes really just seem out of reach, or if you've tried some of those and find yourself at the same place, it may be time to consider medication or hormone therapy and that's okay too!

"Is my low desire hormonal or due to medications I'm using?"

If you're a grown-up and have sex troubles in a relationship, people scoff: "Hormones? I can't believe that. It must be more about the communication, our relationship, and how we feel about each other!" Hmm . . . That's interesting. Remember those seventeen-year-olds at the movies you saw last week who couldn't keep their hands off each other? Was your reaction, "Wow, they must be having deep and meaningful conversations?"

Although we know instinctively that hormones are the driving factor behind libido in young people, we somehow forget that as we get older. Low testosterone has a significant impact on a woman's desire, as do other hormones, such as estrogen[5] and prolactin.[6] That's why you saw those kids and thought, "Wow, those hormones must be raging!"

If your hormones are low, it will be very, very difficult to make up the missing points in other areas. You really need those points!

Similarly, I can't tell you the number of patients who come in and report their libido started flagging about six months after going on the pill, then insist it's not the problem. "It can't be that," they say. "I asked my doctor, and he says it's not possible." Oh, yeah? Well, how about this. Stop the birth control for six months, and we'll see.

If you suspect a medication is affecting your sex life, trust yourself. Drugs can have a significant impact on sexual desire, for good and for bad. Hormonal birth control and SSRIs (antianxiety meds and antidepressants) are the most common culprits. But, as I tell my patients on a daily basis, every woman is a person, not a statistic. If you notice a drop in desire after starting a drug, make sure to find out if the drug is creating the problem—and find a doctor who takes your concerns seriously.

Chapters 9–11 talk about medications; you'll need the help of a medical practitioner for these approaches, and understanding what's happening before you go will be enormously helpful.

"Is my low desire actually a reaction to one or more of the following problems?"

Pain: Here's the thing: if a woman has pain but her libido is still good, she usually finds a way to have sex anyhow. With that in mind, give the pain chapter a review (Chapter 4) and see whether the story checks out.

Problems with arousal: You know what I am going to say here, don't you? Go back and read the chapter on arousal (Chapter 5). Then, find the chapters that outline the places to get points: hormones (Chapter 10), medications and procedures (Chapter 11), lifestyle shifts (Chapter 19), and relationship fixes (Chapters 15, 17, and 18).

Problems with orgasm: Is your lack of orgasm affecting your low desire? This is a very common concern. If you are getting turned on but don't get to orgasm, it can absolutely create low desire. But if that is the case you need to dig deep on orgasm—in the orgasm chapter (Chapter 6).

"Are there drugs that could help my low desire?"

Yes, there are. And guess what? I have a whole chapter on that as well (Chapter 9).

"WHERE'D THE OTHER PART OF ME GO?": MARILYN'S STORY

Marilyn is a fifty-three-year-old woman who went into menopause abruptly at forty-six, when her period disappeared and never returned. Even though she had once had a robust sex life, gradually she began to feel sexually numb, dry, and neutered.

When she remarried at age fifty, her new husband was patient and loving. He would gingerly initiate sex, hoping Marilyn would show some interest, but she felt she just couldn't fake it anymore. It was upsetting, but, it seemed, they would have to accept it. Then, she read an article about testosterone treatment in the *New York Times* and a lightbulb went on in her head. With some trepidation, she looked for a medical center that would treat her with hormones. Her husband was skeptical, but, Marilyn told us later, she just wasn't ready to give up sex without a fight.

She shook her head in frustration as she talked to us.

"This is making me absolutely nuts," she says. "I LOVED sex. I had a great sex drive. Even when my last marriage was falling apart, I was having decent sex with him. Then about three years ago, it was like I dried up. Nothing is working right anymore. I couldn't care less if I ever have sex again. When we do have sex, I have to work at keeping my focus. And my orgasms? Ha! Not even worth the effort. I feel awful for my new husband. He's great. I adore him and he's incredibly understanding and patient, but he's a little disappointed.

"And you know what? I'M DISAPPOINTED. Here I am, sharing my life with a great guy I find very attractive. And I am so shut down. Where'd the other part of me go? I want to want him. I want to have great sex with him. I want him to get to see the terrific sexy part of me that I loved so much. I used to be so sexual. I want it back!"

I spent some time talking to Marilyn. Her relationship, while not perfect, did not seem to be the problem. She was clearly not depressed, and her blood work showed no significant problems.

Her testosterone level, however, was really low. We obviously had no way of knowing what her testosterone level had been ten years ago when her libido was good, but it seemed reasonable to start her on a regimen of testosterone. She had all the hallmarks of someone with a hormone problem: a stable and good relationship, no extraordinary stressors, and a significant decline in desire.

Eighteen months after starting hormone therapy, Marilyn was back: "I had sex with my husband three times in one weekend—all on my own initiative—and it was wonderful. I don't feel thirty again, but I sure feel like I'm forty! My husband is thrilled, and I feel like myself again. I learned that it takes time for your brain and body to kick in, but the months of hormone therapy were worth it. I always had faith this treatment would work, and I am glad I stuck with it. Listen to your own body!"

Marilyn, I couldn't have said it better myself.

Want some of these points back? See Chapters 8–11 and 15–19.

PART III

THE SOLUTIONS!

CHAPTER 8

THE QUICK FIX
Small Ideas That Allow for Big Changes

+80 points . . . temporarily

Addressing:

Primary: Pain, Arousal, Orgasm, and Desire

This chapter is intended to help you immediately, today, with some *short*, easy-to-access solutions, with many points, quickly. It includes some of the best techniques I've used most successfully over the years with some of my patients. The ideas in this chapter may seem deceptively simple; some might seem more complicated. Some of these solutions will hold you in good stead over time and you will continue to use them even if you find other, long-term solutions. Some of them may fall away as the situation improves, but you should start here if you just want to cry and scream "HELP ME!"

A word of caution: These "quick fixes" might not solve all, or even part of the underlying problem you have identified, and they may be temporary, but they are intended to get your sex life back on track, in the moment. That is, if you are having pain and you follow my advice to stop having intercourse, it obviously isn't solving the underlying problem of the pain and you will still need to figure out a long-term solution. But these quick fixes are intended to take the pressure off immediately to help you have a vibrant and active sex life, even while you are solving your longer-term issue.

TALK TO YOUR PARTNER

If you have a partner, talk to them before you put any of these temporary fixes in place. In many cases, the stress put on a relationship because of a dysfunctional sex life can be extreme. And I'm guessing that your partner is as unhappy as you are. There are a number of reasons it is key to have this discussion:

- You want them to know that the state of your sex life is bothering you as well as them and that you are taking steps to fix the problem.
- You want them to be a part of the solution.
- You don't want to spring new ideas, solutions, or devices on them without having an open conversation about what is really going on.
- If it's easier to have your partner read this part of the book, go for it. Sometimes you can rely on my help to explain something that can be pretty difficult to explain.

PAIN

First up: If You Are Having Pain with Intercourse . . . STOP!

I can't tell you how many patients I have who have intercourse even though it hurts. So, before I say anything else, if intercourse hurts, stop having intercourse. Period.

Here's why it's a bad idea to keep having intercourse when it hurts:

- It hurts! You should treat yourself better than to continually cause yourself pain.
- It might exacerbate the problem. If there is an infection, or even just skin irritation, why would you want to continue to irritate the area? If the muscles are tight, the fear will have you tensing up even more and creating more of a problem.

- You will be creating a link in your head between sex and pain. And that is never a good thing. Your body has a strong memory, some even say "the body keeps the score." If it knows that sexual activity will lead to pain, it sets up a Pavlovian reaction and that creates all kinds of secondary problems: Your body tenses up instinctively, you start experiencing stress with sex, and you become avoidant. Often the secondary fear does even more damage than the initial pain did.

Now, please bear in mind that doesn't mean you need to stop having sex. It just means you have to have a different kind of sex for a little while.

Sex Does Not Equal Intercourse. Intercourse Does Not Equal Sex.

This is a good time to point out that sex and intercourse are not synonymous, despite how often our society says that it is. Oral sex is sex. Manual sex (using your hands) is sex. Rubbing your body against each other until you have orgasms is sex. There are so many and varied ways to have sex that taking intercourse out of the mix should not, theoretically, kill your entire sex life.

It used to confuse me that women who had pain with intercourse stopped having sex altogether. Then, I realized how many couples base their sex life on intercourse. Taking it out of their repertoire feels unnatural. For some women, it was their favorite way to have sex. For some, it is the partner's favorite way to have sex. Some say that when they start to have other kinds of sex, their partners naturally gravitate toward intercourse and then they get stuck "trying again." Some women talk about enjoying nonintercourse sex but always feeling guilty or "less than" when they can't seem to have vaginal intercourse. They will speak of not feeling like a "normal woman."

Sex may—and often does—include intercourse. Intercourse can include both vaginal and anal intercourse and is often a part of sex. These distinctions have an impact on our feelings about ourselves.

But the idea that sex has to include intercourse can lead to a very boring sex life.

First, when we use the words *sex* and *intercourse* synonymously, we are not so subtly putting down oral sex, anal sex, manual sex (and any kind of sex you can think of using ten fingers, toes, feathers, or lips). By calling them just foreplay, we are saying that those are not the real deal.

But if every time you have sex, you feel that the culmination is always putting item A in slot B, it can take away a lot of the fun and spontaneity. There is always a temptation to just "get to it" and everything else becomes an unnecessary add-on. It can cause you and your partner to feel that you didn't "really" have sex last night when you had a wonderful session of lovemaking where both of you felt great and came to orgasm with the other's hand, mouth, or other body part or toy.

Also, not everyone loves vaginal intercourse best. For some women, sex feels different at different times in their life. Some may experience pain or discomfort with intercourse, or some may feel bored with intercourse in a long-term relationship. Men, as they get older, may sometimes need more and stronger stimulation than a vagina can give them. Are we telling a couple that has great oral or manual sex two times a week that they are not having sex?

Couples whose sexual relationship is largely based on intercourse look at me funny when I suggest having nonintercourse sex. They are not even sure what I mean. Didn't you just say to stop having sex?

No. I did not say to stop having sex. I said to stop having intercourse. There are a million types of sex you can have that don't involve penetration of the penis in the vagina, or penetration at all, for that matter. And while you are working on getting rid of the pain in your vagina, it's more important than ever to keep having sex! Why?

- Having regular sexual activity is good for your relationships and your happiness.
- Not having sex often starts to create emotional and physical distance between you and your partner.
- Not having sex makes it much harder to reconnect when you fix the pain.
- Sexual activity tends to be cyclical. When you are having regular sex, it's much easier to just shift the way you are having sex.
- If you aren't having any type of sex, it becomes much more complicated to go back to having sex.

In the meantime, speak with your partner and figure out what ways the two of you can continue to have sex, in a way that feels good and fun to you both.

There are so many ways to have sex that do not include intercourse, so if you are having pain, sit down with your partner. Talk about it. And make a list of alternative sexual activities that don't hurt, but feel good and bring on orgasms for both of you. If your partner is male and complains that intercourse is his preferred way of having sex, that's too bad. I hope he prefers to have sex a second-best way rather than not have sex at all. If not . . . then there are bigger issues that need to be discussed.

Stop thinking of oral sex (using your mouth) and manual sex (using your hands) as foreplay. It's not. It's sex. So, sit down and make some rules. And use any variation of the following conversation:

"Honey, I've been thinking about how little sex we've been having recently. And I feel bad about it, but the truth is every time we have intercourse it hurts. And it's not getting better. But I don't want to whine about it or complain about it, so I just tense up and bear it, but that approach is not working. It's just making things worse, I think. So, I've been thinking, can we schedule sex without intercourse for the next two months or so while I start looking around for a doctor or physical therapist who may be able to help? I really miss having a sex life with you and I think if I know, at the outset, that we won't be trying to have intercourse but will be doing other things, I won't be scared of the pain and I will be happy to go back to having sex with you."

"I know I've been hesitant to give you oral sex, but I've been looking into ways that I can do that. Also, I've bought some new lube that I can use on you with my hands, and a nifty device we can try, called a sleeve, which is supposed to feel like a vagina. I'm sure it doesn't, but what the hell, let's just try?"

You need to figure out a way to continue having sex on a regular basis but not have intercourse. It's as simple as that. And honestly, as complicated as that. Because sometimes, my patients feel guilty and confused. They also sometimes think that "working through the pain" is the way to go. And sometimes, their partners make them feel that if they are not having intercourse, "it's not really sex." So, if you are struggling with pain, I deeply urge you not to give up on your sex life but to focus on the myriad other ways to give and receive pleasure from your partner. Address the problem head on. And then head to the bedroom.

AROUSAL/ORGASM

If you are having trouble getting turned on or having an orgasm, there is no easier and no more straightforward solution than finding a good, strong, vibrator. And Chapter 14 should give you all the information you need to get going on a vibrator purchase.

Here's the deal: Many women just need more stimulation than they can get from a hand, a mouth, or a penis, and a vibrator can provide that. That doesn't mean that a vibrator is going to be the end solution. It is possible that over time you will need to take a good hard look at your hormones (Chapter 10) or at your medications (Chapter 11), or at the fantasies you may or may not be having (Chapter 16). But in the meantime, take a shortcut and choose a good strong vibrator that will make it easier for you to get the stimulation you need.

Contrary to popular notion, vibrators aren't useful just for solo masturbation; they are often used in partner sex as well, either before intercourse, after intercourse, or instead of intercourse.

Some women feel that there is something "fake" or "unnatural" about a vibrator. I don't have a great deal of patience for that. Is there something unnatural about a guy who needs to take Viagra to get strong erections? Not in my book. He just has blood flow issues. Or let's take the example of vision issues. Is using eyeglasses unnatural? There is absolutely nothing wrong with using mechanics or gadgets to make things "work better." And vibrators are in the same category.

Here's a word of caution. If you are thinking of getting a vibrator, dig into Chapter 14 so that you educate yourself. But if you are going after a vibrator because you are finding orgasms elusive, there are two particular versions of vibrators I recommend:

- If you used to have orgasms but they seem to have gone on a permanent vacation, you probably want to find a fairly sizable and strong chargeable vibrator. Forget the battery-operated cute, small ones. They won't be helpful. You need strength and consistency. Go for one that looks like a small handheld microphone with a head that is the size of a tennis ball or larger. There are any number of models like this but do a quick search and you won't have trouble finding one. If you are unsure, the bigger the better.
- If you have never had an orgasm, you might want to try one of the strong ones described above, but you also might want to try one of the new suction models. These are more like the size of your cupped hand and they have a head inserted in them that includes a suction. These vibrators are much more gentle than their big kahuna friends, but they have a subtle way

of coaxing an orgasm out of women who haven't been able to climax before.

So, go take a better look at Chapter 14 on vibrators and see whether you can get over any discomfort or embarrassment you may have. This may be an easy solution for managing the problem right now, while you look for other points that may take longer to access.

LOW DESIRE

If you came into my office and said that you are dragging yourself to have sex and hating every miserable moment of it, or you said you hadn't had sex in a year or more, there would be many more questions to ask. I would want to find out whether you and your partner were having difficulties (either prior to this problem or as a result of this problem). I would want to figure out whether you were depressed. I would want to find out what medications you might be on that would be affecting your sex drive. I would want to look at your hormone profile. I would want to understand your self-image and what you thought about sex and whether this had ever been any different or was always like this. But one of the first, most generic questions I would ask would be:

In addition to sex, are you avoiding touching your partner in general? Are you not kissing or hugging or cuddling or snuggling because you are afraid that your partner will see that as an invitation for sex, or even just open up the door so that they will want to have sex when you do that? One of the most heart-wrenching sights is a woman sitting across from me, sobbing, because she feels so guilty that she has not only been avoiding sex, but she has been avoiding any type of physical intimacy as well because she is scared it will "lead to sex." This is such a common syndrome that I feel like it should have its own name. But it doesn't. At least, not yet. The level of guilt and shame these women carry is almost unbearable. And the first thing I will do with these women is suggest scheduling "not-sex."

Scheduling Not-Sex: While You're Figuring Out Your Low Desire

Sex therapists are famous for telling couples to schedule sex to solve months-long sex droughts. And it's not a bad idea. But it is only half the equation. The other half is *scheduling when not to have sex.*

Why?

Because while scheduling sex helps the partner who is despondent at never having sex, it doesn't address the low-desire partner's needs. So, while Sally, who never wants to have sex, now, upon the suggestion of her sex therapist, agrees to have sex once a week with her husband, she finds herself in a bind worse than when she started. She is having sex once a week, and her partner, who is thrilled that she is "back," starts to assume that since it was so good yesterday, they should try again today. Sally is now a combination of pissed off and guilty. "We just HAD sex!" she thinks. "There is no way I am going to kiss him when he gets home today. He's going to think I'm up for having sex again."

One of the things I have found to be true is that when there are clear and specific times when sex is *off the table entirely*, the guilt and the self-blame dissolves, and the low-desire partner is much more open to planned sporadic sexual activity. Additionally, and just as important, it frees up the low-desire partner to be fun, playful, and connected in all kinds of physical ways without the stress of having sex hanging over her head. Often, the partners of women with low desire will mourn the lack of sex. But in addition, they will talk poignantly about the fact that not only are they not having sex, but all physical connection is gone as well. Their wife, or girlfriend, no longer kisses, caresses, or snuggles with them. Sometimes partners feel the loss of this even more acutely than the absence of sex.

So, here's how you do it. As you're figuring out the low-desire issue, together, come up with a schedule of times when you will have sex. Usually, this will be once a week. Sometimes, it's twice a month. It has to be a frequency that you, the low-desire partner, feel can be maintained without feeling resentful. Then, set a *specific time* aside for sexual activity, such as Sunday morning first thing, or Friday afternoon after work, or after the kids are in bed. At those times, you will commit to having sex with your partner in as positive a way as possible. You won't wait to be asked, cajoled, wined, and dined. Your partner will not have to dance around the subject carefully, hoping you will get the hint and not bite their head off. You will be in it as fully as you can possibly be. If for some reason the specific time that you both set aside will not work for logistical reasons (e.g., your partner has the flu or you are away on a business trip) you, the lower-desire partner, *will have the full responsibility* for rescheduling another **specific** time in its place.

And then, when you both have agreed to have some type of sexual activity at that specific time, you concomitantly agree *not to have sex at any other time*! During the rest of your set time period, there will *be no expectation* of sexual activity. Even if the low-desire partner cuddles, kisses, snuggles, climbs naked into bed, and spoons, their partner will understand that it is not an invitation to engage in sex. It is amazing to see how liberating this process can be. The only exception is if the low-desire partner says the words (verbally and aloud): "Hey, actually I'm in the mood. Let's have sex now."

Here's what I see when couples schedule the on and off times:

- It reassures the partner who wants and needs more sex that they will get it, and tells them when. It may not be as often as they want, but it won't be never. The relief in knowing that sex is not gone forever, nor subject to what seems like the inexplicable whims of their partner, act like magic. Their partner feels less stressed-out, less irritable, less lonely, and more patient and loving.
- It breaks the guilt cycle for the low-desire partner. So many women tell me that they walk around with a ticking clock in their head: "It's been three days since we've had sex. It's been a week since we've had sex. Oh, no. It's been two weeks since we've had sex. How long can I draw this out? Maybe I should

initiate sex tonight? Maybe tomorrow?" Lots of guilt, resentment, and other emotional dark clouds start to build. Often, when a woman knows she's having sex at a set time, it takes away the bad feelings. The sex date has parameters. It's limited. This stops the ticking clock.

- Scheduling time off lets the low-desire partner go back to being physical and demonstrative. Gestures like kisses or snuggling or hugs can happen again when there's no fear they'll be misunderstood as invitation. Not-sex allows couples to return to physical contact and intimacy they may not have experienced in years.
- Finally, there are times when "not having sex" becomes a habit. Changing habits, as we all know, can be very difficult. Having a scheduled time for sex may help couples rekindle their sex life on a new footing.

For this to work, both partners have to sign on and be absolutely vigilant about maintaining their boundaries and responsibilities. If one partner does not fulfill their part of the bargain, the entire enterprise becomes useless. If, for example, the low-desire partner acts resentful and put upon when it's time to have sex at the designated time, their partner will likely feel betrayed and abandoned, and become angry, hurt, or resentful. By the same token, if the higher-desire partner makes a move to have sex at a nonscheduled time, the low-desire partner will lose trust that sex is off the table at the times they have agreed upon. They will not believe that they can be physical and loving without its leading to sex, and they will likely revert to their inability or unwillingness to do so. I've created a "cheat sheet" for you to give to your partner, and you can find it at the end of the book (see Appendix I).

The Chicken or the Egg?

Here's the complication. You haven't had sex in (fill in the blank: two months, six months, two years, five years). Now what? You can't even imagine discussing this with your partner. Thinking about it makes you want to cry. You feel like you are a lost cause. There is no way to get sex back on the table. Worse still, you wonder if you even want to make things better. You wonder whether you are so "out of love" that it feels a bit ludicrous to be trying to repair your sex life. "Maybe the bottom line is that I'm out of love with this person or I'm just not attracted to them anymore." What then?

Here's what you are really asking: Does a good sex life improve a relationship or does a better relationship encourage a good sex life? That is the million-dollar question. The answer I see every day in our center is "both."

The idea that sex creates greater intimacy gets lost when we only think about intimacy encouraging sex. There's even a subtle bias against using sex to create intimacy. "She only slept with him to get him off her case." "I'm not gonna have sex if I don't feel close to him." "I can't believe she had sex when she wasn't in the mood."

Our society has a crazy bias against physical communication, whereas verbal communication is lauded. If you have fallen in love because you talk for hours, that's good. If you have fallen in love because you like the way they kiss, that's superficial. Talking to work out problems is considered the gold standard. You can spend a year in therapy talking about issues and getting nowhere, but that is okay. Running a marathon or punching a pillow, less so. That's why so many couples therapists get away with seeing clients for years and never discussing their sex life. They assume (incorrectly, by the way) that if they improve the relationship, the sex will follow naturally. You should be aware that there are many couples therapists who are not comfortable dealing with sex. They don't mean badly, but a couple whose major issue might really and truly be sexual, might sit and spend half a year talking about their parents, their communication, their abandonment issues . . . and then they quit and are worse off than when they started because now they think they've already "tried the therapy route." Don't fall into that trap!

Talking is all great and good. I LOVE talking. Just ask my husband and kids. But talking is just one avenue of a relationship, a truly important one. But it's not an avenue to fixing all of your problems. In my experience, it's only a small part of fixing your sex life.

Thank goodness, the psychological community is starting to understand that the mind and body are intrinsically linked and each powerfully affects the other, and is embracing somatic therapy (therapy that uses both psychotherapy and physical movement), mindfulness, and meditation.

Perhaps we should be more open to using sex to help heal a relationship. Sometimes a behavioral answer can address a problem more directly and quickly than long-term analysis. If we start to think of sex not only as a means of expressing intimacy when it already exists, but instead as a tool to help reintroduce or re-create intimacy it might give us a new, more practical framework. What follows, as a result, can be more intimacy and better communication.

So, before you are quick to dismiss the idea of sex because you are not "in the mood," or things have been tense with you and your partner recently, perhaps consider the idea that sex may help heal and build the intimacy between the two of you.

Here are some steps I suggest taking to start this conversation:

- Set up a time to talk. Don't spring it on your partner. You've had time to think about this and mull it over. So should they. Do not talk about it in the bedroom. Do not talk about it immediately before or after you have had sex, and definitely do not talk about it after you have just rejected your partner . . . again. Maybe, one night alone after dinner, say, "I'd like to talk about sex . . . and the fact that we aren't having any . . . can we set up a time to talk about it?"
- When you do talk about it, try very hard not to blame anyone but to keep the tone neutral. Try to describe how you are feeling about it and be honest (as kindly as you can) as to why you

think there might be a problem. "I know this is a complicated problem, but I feel smothered/creeped out by your neediness/bothered by how hard it is for you to come/angry at your expectations/whiplashed by how fast you turn around from work to sex/I honestly believe this is a physiological problem I'm having and not much to do with the relationship."

- Put some clear and practical suggestions on the table as to how you might begin to fix the problem. "I am making an appointment with a doctor. I'd like you to make an appointment with a doctor. I want to schedule 'not-sex,' so let's read this chapter together. I want to consider using a vibrator."
- And keep the following in mind:
  - Make it clear that you don't think this will be a problem that is solved overnight.
  - Try not to get defensive.
  - Try not to be offensive.
  - Listen. A lot.

Sexual problems are complicated. And often they seem insurmountable when you are living them. But the good news is that often they are shockingly easy to turn around. Once the downward spiral is broken and the wheels start turning in the other direction, you would be amazed at how fast things can improve. You need points. You need them quickly. And you can get a whole boatload fast with these suggestions. They probably won't raise your point threshold permanently by themselves, but they should provide a good fast influx to start turning the cycle around.

Now, go ahead and use the following chapters to take a deep dive into finding yourself more points.

CHAPTER 9

THE DRUG WARS

Why Big Pharma Might Not Be All Bad

S ome women come into my office and tell me immediately, "I'll do anything. Just don't give me any drugs."

This puts me in a funny bind. On the one hand, I get it. We live in a society where people seem more inclined to pop a pill than to ask what's contributing to the problem. When there's an underlying problem, a pill can simply cover it up. Take pain medication, such as Tylenol or Excedrin. When something hurts, you may want to try to see why, before you simply cut the pain receptors. One podcast made me laugh out loud when a contributor said, "Taking pain medication when you don't know what the problem is, is kind of like cutting the wires to your battery when your 'service engine' button lights up."

But there are physiologic problems that need physiologic responses: from stretching to exercise to, yes, medication. I am often amused when things doctors assumed were psychological are revealed to be primarily physiological problems. Take male erectile dysfunction, or impotence. Twenty-five years ago, if you could not achieve or maintain an erection, your family doctor would have sent you to a psychologist to "understand" what was going on. You could have spent two years talking until you were blue in the face, but if the problem is blood flow to your penis or the ability of your muscles to hold onto blood, talking doesn't help!

Take PMS. For years, doctors said that there was no such thing: women were just "moody." It was only when we accepted there was a powerful hormonal component to PMS that we could help women who were suffering for no reason.

When discussing sexual problems, both doctors and therapists persist in defining issues as either "in the body" or "in the head." A firestorm ignited in 2015 when the FDA approved the first drug for female sexual dysfunction, Addyi. Doctors were skeptical that the drug would help, and therapists threw up their arms in disgust at the "medicalization" of female sexuality. In other words, doctors couldn't see beyond handing the patient a pill, and the therapists couldn't see the value of one.

But all—and I mean *all*—of our current research supports the idea that the physiological and the psychological work in tandem. One of my all-time favorite studies shows that when men become caregivers to their children, their testosterone levels actually drop.[1] The line between "psychological" and "physiological" is more of a handshake, and such binary thinking is ridiculously antiquated. This failure to work together hurts our patients. Once we understand the physical components, we have a much more real and deep understanding of the problem.

When mental health professionals don't like sexual health medicines, they point to a drug's relatively low (although still significant) success rate in trials. And of course, they are right. But what they fail to realize is that drug trials usually prohibit simultaneous talk or behavioral therapy. Physicians also fail to understand that, even when extremely effective drugs are prescribed, behaviors may need to change for it to work.

I often give Grand Rounds—talks to physicians and nurse practitioners—in hospitals. And when I talk about treating low desire with testosterone, doctors sometimes tell me, "I've tried it. It doesn't work."

I look at them with a mixture of horror and amusement. In their lexicon, I know "trying it" means giving the woman a prescription and sending her home. There is no follow-up, no understanding of behaviors that can make real and lasting changes. Determining that a drug "doesn't work" when it's not administered effectively is like performing surgery and not sending the patient for follow-up care or physical therapy.

On the other side are my colleagues the therapists. They are so busy putting down the drug companies that they won't even consider that medications can provide us with a leg up in our work. My colleagues have a knee-jerk reaction: it hasn't worked, it won't work, the side effects are too problematic, it "masks" the real problem. Some therapists argue that women's sexual dysfunction is a myth created by the media and that the search for medical solutions is merely a thinly veiled way for the pharmaceutical companies to fleece innocent and gullible women. Hearing that makes me crazy!

The truth is, there is little evidence that sex therapy alone has any significant and lasting impact for low desire. When a woman's body is fighting her interest in sex, all the techniques in the world—slowing things down, sensate focus, fantasizing, sexy lingerie—have only limited impact. But in these conversations, there is no recognition that drugs could make us able to do our job better and more effectively.

I have worked for many years giving testosterone to women with low libido. We treat them with hormones or other medications *at the same time* that we provide sexuality counseling and behavioral and psychological support for these changes. And I can see the powerful results when used in combination, much more powerful than when each is used alone.

It is important for sex therapists to acknowledge that the working of the body is relevant and critical to changes in behavior. And medical doctors need to appreciate that medical interventions, while often significant, can be dramatically enhanced by working in tandem with therapists. A surgeon wouldn't send a patient home after surgery without very specific instructions, specific exercises, and physical therapy. And sexual health practitioners should understand that drugs may be just a first step in treatment. The beneficiaries would be our patients.

Now, let's talk about trust.

So, those big bad pharmaceutical companies are indeed account-able to their shareholders. Profit and share-price are the motives for making a product that works and will sell to a large patient popula-tion. No question.

But what if the motivation for studying a solution for millions of women *is* profit? Personally, I don't really care what their motives are, as long as they are working on the problem. If Big Pharma is trying to produce a drug that may help low desire or arousal, good for them! This may also be good for some my patients, which is the point, isn't it?

Remember, whether you're a consumer or a patient, you are an in-telligent and responsible person and you can evaluate all of the treat-ment options with your unique understanding of your own needs, and with an eye toward efficacy and safety and effort. The only ques-tions you should ask yourself when you are considering any treatment are: will it work and is it safe? After that, the next question can be: how long will it take? (The adult version of "Are we there yet?") Then, you can make an informed and useful decision on what treatment modalities you want to use.

As you look through these next two chapters, keep an open mind. Understanding the utility of medicines can be extraordinarily useful in building up a point profile, especially when your life is pulling you in ten different directions and time-intensive treatments don't make sense. There will also be times when drug use isn't possible or recom-mended, or when you have adverse reactions. Then, you will need to garner points using other methods.

Now that I gave you a too-long lecture about medicine and sex, I will try to outline a practical approach. There are medications that can help you and add points to your sexual profile. There are medica-tions that can get in the way and take away points from your sexual profile. And a word of caution: The next two chapters outline typi-cal medications, including how they may hurt your point profile and how they may help. But please remember, they include the drugs and the reactions that we typically see. You may be different. Just because most women find that they have a harder time having orgasms when they are on Effexor, you may not! You are an individual, with your own individual responses. You are not a number on a chart. So, look through the next two chapters. See whether you can find some places to take back points or maybe get some new ones. And then speak to your physician.

CHAPTER 10

HORMONES

It's Not Your Head, It's Your Bloodstream

> *+80 points*
> *Addressing:*
> *Primary: Pain, Arousal, Desire*
> *Secondary: Orgasm*

We don't like attributing our sexual functioning to hormones. Instead, we'll say, "It's all about the relationship," or "It's all about confidence." We tell ourselves that if we don't want sex, it's psychological or emotional. We tell ourselves we aren't concentrating enough on the erotic, that we're not knowledgeable enough, or that we're not making enough time for our partners.

Because they are invisible, we treat hormones as if they don't exist. Trust me—it's not "all in your head." We are just starting to understand our hormones and how powerfully they can affect our interest in sex and our ability to respond to sexual activities. What is it that makes us WANT to concentrate more on sex? What makes us want to find out more, want to explore more, and want to make time for sex? *What puts sex into our head?* Plain and simple, hormones exert a powerful control over our sex life.

In fact, hormones have such a significant impact on who we are and how we react to things that when they are in the wrong ratio, low, or even missing, everything—*including* sex—is thrown off balance. We can get anxious and moody, depressed and lethargic, or overly agitated. We can experience significant weight gain or loss—muscle changes and skin changes. We can grow too much, or too little. And we can lose our sex drive—or develop a massive one.

As kids go through puberty, we *expect* them to suddenly develop an interest in sex. But what exactly is puberty? It's an increase in those hormones that make you interested in sex! When we see a gangly adolescent boy ogling another teenager on the street, we even say it: "His hormones are raging." We understand that in teenagers, hormones are the engine that powers the sex drive.

But somehow, as soon as it comes to understanding the adult libido, we change our tune. Now, it's all about relationships, conversations, and sexy underwear. Don't get me wrong. Our relationship, our confidence, and even sexy underwear can play an important part. And exactly how hormones work on the brain, how they interact with one another, and what specific quantities people need to "work right" is still being studied; those of us in the field of sexual health know that without a proper hormonal profile, the odds of sexual problems go way up. Hormones aren't just life-changing when we're a teenager. They have a significant role in our sexual experience throughout our entire adult life, and in my experience, they affect all four quadrants in a powerful way. And that's why I say that they are responsible for a whopping 80 points when we're talking about the 100-point threshold. If your hormones are really low, it's unlikely that any amount of therapy or behavior modification can fix that.

Take two girls, both growing up in a firmly Catholic family in which parents make it clear that they must wait until marriage for sex. One of them responds by dutifully listening, holding off on sexual activity until she is in a serious relationship at age twenty-four. The other? She starts masturbating at age ten and is climbing out the proverbial window to meet her boyfriend at fifteen. A logical explanation? Biology.

Hormones can also cause other, less-expected problems. If you are having pain, it may be due to the changes wrought by hormonal birth control. How? Synthetic estrogen, which is in most birth controls, often stops your body from creating its own estrogen and inhibits it from making testosterone. Oral contraceptives can increase the SHBG (sex hormone–binding globulin) quite dramatically. The SHBG binds to testosterone and estrogen, holding it hostage in your bloodstream, and not letting it get out of the bloodstream and into your cells, where it does its magic. One of our nurse practitioners used to explain SHBG to patients as a Pac-Man, running around your bloodstream and gobbling up your testosterone and estrogen. One result is that your vagina, which is extraordinarily sensitive to hormonal changes and imbalance, can dry up, or become paper thin.

Desire, arousal, and orgasm are similarly connected to low hormones. As they head into menopause, many women start to feel changes in their sexual responses that can be linked to their changing hormones.[1] They are no longer interested in sex. They can't get aroused. And when they can, there is a significant change in their orgasms. In most cases, when you give women back what their body used to have, their sexual experience improves. Voilà: the hormone solution.

"I WAS AMAZED IT COULD MAKE SUCH A DIFFERENCE": DIANA'S STORY

A forty-six-year-old stay-at-home mother of three children, Diana smiles easily and plays with her red ponytail when she gets nervous. And, she tells me, for many years, she has suffered from a "total lack of desire" for her husband, Victor. She never had a problem having orgasms. But "getting into" sex has been a challenge. "I love him," she says. "He's a great guy. But I just wanted to get it over and done with."

She can't remember a time when she felt differently: "I've never been a really sexual person to begin with. I'm kind of prudish. Whenever girls at college started talking about sex, I would just sit and listen. Everyone else seemed more interested and more fascinated by sex than I was."

Victor tried to understand, but he felt the problem was that she wasn't attracted to him. They compromised: they would "do it" once a week. She complied, without enthusiasm, and, over the years, sex became an almost insurmountable barrier between them. Diana feared it would end her marriage—and that there was nothing she could do about it.

At our office, a blood test revealed that Diana had a low testosterone level. We prescribe testosterone gel, which she would apply each evening to the inside of her leg, and then decreased the dose of the antidepressant she was already taking.

The change in her libido was quickly apparent.

"It's been very different," Diana says now. "I didn't think this would do anything, and I was amazed that it could make such a difference. I don't think women understand or know that. Before getting treatment, I'd cringe every time my husband touched me. Now I'm enjoying it more," she says. "Having sex with Victor once or twice a week is easy for me now."

And Victor, she says, "Doesn't have resentment built up anymore. Now he feels like I'm trying to make things work. It's amazing to think that just that little stuff I'm doing makes such a difference." Now, Diana even initiates sex with her husband, which she admits she never did before. On a recent vacation, they made love "three or four times in four days!" For just about the first time, "I felt like it," Diana says.

SO, ABOUT THESE HORMONES

The hormones that seem to have the most effect on your sex life are testosterone, DHEA-S, estrogen, and progesterone.

Testosterone and DHEA-S

We think of testosterone as being a male hormone because men have a lot of it. Testosterone production in the female body is about twenty times less than in a male body, but it is still a necessary element.[2] It plays a vital role in your health and well-being. As the research in the field grows, we are understanding how central it is to female libido.[3]

There are endless arguments about how to best "give" testosterone to women. When I started in this field, twenty years ago, physicians used an over-the-counter product called DHEA-S (dehydroepi-androsterone sulfate). It is a hormone produced in various parts of both men and women's bodies, including the testicles, ovaries, and brain, but it's primarily produced in the adrenal glands, small glands above the kidney that produce many hormones.

Once in the bloodstream, some DHEA-S is converted into tes-tosterone, some into progesterone, and some into estrogen. So, es-sentially, we weren't giving women testosterone, we were giving them the "precursor": the hormone that, once in their body, is converted into testosterone. Giving DHEA-S felt safer than giving straight tes-tosterone. It was, and is, sold in nutritional supplement stores and in your local pharmacy. Because it is classified as a nutritional supple-ment and not a drug, it isn't FDA-regulated, and you would need to take extremely large amounts to significantly change your testoster-one levels. And that is the precise reason it also often wasn't so help-ful for women. DHEA-S is subtle, slow, and gentle. The quantities prescribed often weren't enough to help significantly, or would take forever to produce effects.

Although it may not make sense to use DHEA-S as a means of boosting testosterone, it does sometimes make sense to use a DHEA-S supplement to counter the effects of other hormonal prob-lems. For example, when problems start with drugs that throw off women's normal hormone production, such as birth control pills, or there has been a life-changing event, such as pregnancy, that inter-feres with a woman's regular hormone profile, we have found that in these situations DHEA-S can be helpful and can add points for women because it converts into many different hormones (testos-terone, estrogen, and progesterone). While the body's hormones are trying to straighten themselves out, DHEA-S can give them a point boost quickly and easily. If you do decide to take DHEA-S, even though you can buy it over the counter, you should consider consulting a medical provider so that you can have regular blood checks to make sure that your other hormones aren't going too high.

But if you are really after a higher level of testosterone, DHEA-S is probably not the answer. Usually women need to have their testosterone supplemented directly.

HOW MUCH TESTOSTERONE SHOULD YOU HAVE?

That is a great question, but not a particularly easy one to answer. Very little data are available on "normal" levels for women. When women tell me, "My doctor checked my testosterone level and it was normal," I say, "Normal for what? For not being dead?" "Normal" testosterone levels used by general practitioners are calibrated only to assume there's no significant disease state.

It's clear that a woman's body creates significantly less testosterone as she gets older.[4] In men, most testosterone is created in the testes; in women, the ovaries. In both sexes, the rest is created in the adrenal glands. But as women's ovaries start "slowing down," they release fewer eggs and produce less testosterone.

Measuring testosterone is a complicated project. First of all, it is a sensitive test, and many labs are not equipped to do it properly. Second, there are major differences between laboratories. If you have your testosterone checked in two different labs, you get very different results. When you are trying to raise your testosterone levels and you can't tell whether things are actually improving, that can be a problem. To make matters more complicated, your testosterone fluctuates. It's higher in the morning, and up and down during the day.

So, when you are being treated for testosterone, you are looking for a trend, rather than one number. Your practitioner should give you a target range. As long as your blood tests, even if they fluctuate, are moving in the proximity of that range, or increasing slowly into that range as you start treatment, you will know you are on the right track. You are not looking for one magic number. If you come in with your blood testosterone test registering at 10, and, after having your testosterone supplemented, have results trending 35, 22, 57, 40, or 60, you know you are on the right track.

Unfortunately, there is no one right way to tell the exact level that will work for you. I often tell my patients that this is as much an art as a science. But it is important to understand your numbers, make sure that a consistent method is being used to monitor your levels, and work with someone who knows how to evaluate your progress.

Researchers and health-care providers quantify testosterone in different ways. Here are the terms you will likely hear floated around by physicians who are testing your testosterone:

Total testosterone: How much testosterone your bloodstream has in total.

Free androgen index or free testosterone: How much of your testosterone is available for your use. Both of these indexes try to get an understanding of the amount of testosterone that actually makes its way out of the bloodstream and can be used by your body's cells. This number is a result of different calculations that look at your total testosterone in relationship to your SHBG and other proteins that bind the testosterone, keeping it in the bloodstream and making it unavailable for the rest of your body.

We do know that women's testosterone levels drop with age, and are significantly affected by stress, eating disorders, and other life factors.[5] We also know that different women process testosterone differently, although it's not yet clear why. It all comes down to their hormone receptors: with the same quantity of a hormone in their system, one woman can access all of it, whereas another woman might only be able to use half. This second woman will obviously need more testosterone supplementation to end up with the same results.[6]

We already discussed how women with high levels of SHBG in their bloodstream—generally from the pill, but also from aging—can find their testosterone hard to access if they are sensitive to hormonal fluctuations. Don't worry. I'm not trying to do a hatchet job on the pill. For many women (probably the ones with the best receptors), being on the pill and having a high SHBG level doesn't seem to create a significant problem, and for them, birth control pills work effectively without creating additional problems. That's why it's important to work with someone who understands the fluctuations and different ways that they can manifest.

WHEN YOU ARE GIVEN TOO MUCH TESTOSTERONE

One day, a journalist who was doing a piece on low desire and its treatment for a women's magazine called me for a quote. She was writing an article, not only about low desire in general, but about her low desire. And she was exploring testosterone treatment. She was great, funny, smart, and savvy. As we spoke, I liked her more and more. I suggested she come in for an evaluation with us since, honestly, I was a bit skeptical about the treatment plan she had been given. The gynecologist had prescribed a testosterone cream and directed her to rub it into her labia. I was concerned about the location of the application, and that her blood levels weren't being monitored.

When we tested her blood, her total testosterone level was at 500. That might be normal for a man, but it is between four and ten times as high as it should be for a woman, according to *anyone* in the field.[7]

"No wonder I was fantasizing about my old grumpy neighbor," she said, laughing, when we called her with the blood test results. It *was* funny in a way, but I was laughing less. When testosterone gets too high, you start seeing side effects, such as hair growth, male-pattern baldness, or acne. In the long term, these can be irreversible, but fortunately, you have to have been using testosterone for quite a while for them to become permanent. Luckily, the writer had only been on the treatment protocol for a month or two. We significantly modified her treatment, shifting her to a cream that she rubbed on her leg, and we monitored her blood levels every three to four months, to keep an eye on it.

HOW DO YOU "TAKE" TESTOSTERONE?

Testosterone is usually given to you in one of three ways: injections, topicals (gels or creams you rub on your thigh), or pellets that are inserted into the fat of your butt cheek about an inch from the surface.

We are not really fans of the injections because, frankly, who loves injections? And also, the type of testosterone available in injections is not bioidentical. (I explain what bioidentical is at the end of this chapter.) For many years, we worked with topical testosterone, starting women on a dosage approximately one-seventh of the male dosage. However, smearing a dollop of gel on their thighs daily was a pain, and because of that, women weren't always so consistent. It could be hard to tell whether levels weren't rising because women weren't using enough every day, or because they were forgetting to use it more times than they thought.

A few years ago, we started offering testosterone pellet inserts, which give us more consistent results. These Tic Tac–like pellets are inserted under the skin of your butt. The procedure takes about ten minutes, is essentially a painless process, and it lasts three months. Whereas men get as many as twenty inserted, women will usually have one to two pellets inserted.

We are getting really good results with women who use the pellets and are not seeing too many side effects. I'm a big fan of this method, so if you are considering testosterone supplementation, you might want to look into pellet insertion.

If you are wondering about oral testosterone, we do not recommend it for several reasons. First, it is not legal in the United States! Second, it is not currently available as a bioidentical product. Third, oral medication passes first through your liver, which gives that organ a high concentration of testosterone. This actually increases the risk of liver cancer, which is not seen in non-oral administration of testosterone.[8]

In the US, there are currently no FDA-approved products for women. That means that clinicians who prescribe testosterone to women must use, off-label, a product created for men. (Off-label means using a medication outside of what FDA has approved it for. Physicians are allowed to do this, and do this very frequently!)

Estrogen

Estrogen is the basic female sex hormone.[9] It is essential for women's sexual characteristics and their reproductive system. It keeps your brain clear and sharp, your hair shiny, your skin soft and clear, and your bones strong.[10] When your body loses its natural estrogen, all these things change. There are three different types of estrogen in your body:

> **Estradiol**, produced in the ovaries, is the strongest type of estrogen. And while it is the best one to reverse all the effects of lost estrogen, it is also thought to contribute to a number of gynecological problems, including endometriosis, fibroids, and endometrial cancer (if there is not progesterone).
>
> **Estrone** is a weak form of estrogen found in postmenopausal women. If need be, the body can convert estrone to estradiol, and estradiol to estrone.
>
> **Estriol** is the weakest of the estrogens. Pregnancy is the only time at which significant amounts of estriol are made. Estriol cannot be converted to estradiol or estrone.

Estrogen levels fluctuate during the month, and it is essential for fertility. However, by the time a woman hits perimenopause or menopause itself, estrogen drops significantly. There may still be fluctuations, but they will trend lower and lower, until they hit zero.

SPEAKING OF MENOPAUSE

Menopause is a time of significant hormonal changes and often simultaneously of life-stage changes. Sometimes, the two can be hard to separate. If you are married with children, this may be the time when your kids are leaving the house, leaving you and your husband alone. If you work outside the home, you may feel bored, or tired of your job, and yearn for new experiences in your work life. You may be newly caring for aging parents, dealing with your own or your spouse's health issues, and evaluating your finances as you look toward retirement. Overall, you are probably reexamining your life and your priorities. That alone can be crazy making.

As if all that weren't enough, during menopause, your estrogen plummets. Hormonal changes can wreak havoc on body and mind, leaving you feeling tired, foggy, or undesirable.

Does any of this sound familiar?

- Your skin has lost some of its glow.
- Your hair is thinning.
- Your midsection is widening, no matter how much you exercise.
- You are wondering who has run off with a piece of your brain.
- Your sleep is disturbed.
- You are moody. Maybe all the time.
- You're too tired to have sex—maybe because hormonal shifts have left you with no libido.
- Your vaginal lining is dry and thinning, and the muscles and skin tightening.
- Intercourse hurts.

Many, if not all, of these symptoms can now be treated medically. That doesn't mean doctors have always done it correctly. During the 1990s into the mid-aughts, physicians were giving out oral synthetic estrogen like M&M's. Then came a large-scale study that showed potentially additional risk of strokes and heart problems with high dosages of synthetic hormones.[11] That caused the medical community to start treating all estrogen as if it were flammable. Every woman stopped taking estrogen, and no one was prescribed it. There were a lot of miserable women and partners! Neither extreme protocol made sense.

Now, twenty years after that fateful study, we have a better understanding of how terribly flawed that study was, how dramatically skewed the results were, and what is safe and what may not be. Certain types of cancers have been linked to estrogen, and if you have a family history of those types of cancers, estrogen treatment might not be in the cards for you[12] (though you almost always can still take testosterone). But estrogen can be incredibly helpful in terms of keeping your bones from getting brittle, your brain spry, and your hair, skin, and vagina supple.[13] You have a right to be treated with estrogen if you think it is right for you, and I encourage you, if you are not getting good support from your current provider, to find a new one. In the end, it is your body, your choice, and your sex life.

Prescription estrogen is administered in a few different ways: patches, puffers, and rings. You can take estrogen by putting on a tiny patch twice a week, by spritzing it on your skin (with a really powerful "puff" that pushes it through), or even sliding a flexible ring into your vagina for three months. Each has its own advantages and, since no one method of delivery is better than the other, you can choose the best one for you with advice from your health-care provider.[14]

Progesterone

We don't exactly know how progesterone affects your sex life. But we do know now that it is crucial to balance any estrogen you may be taking. Here's how it works: Estrogen signals your body to build up the uterine lining so that when an egg is released, it will have a healthy blood-lined uterus to attach itself to. In premenopausal women who are not taking outside estrogen, toward the end of the cycle, estrogen drops, progesterone goes up, and this signals the woman's body to stop holding onto the uterine lining. Our period is when the lining "sheds" or sloughs off. This is why, when you stop taking birth control pills, you start to bleed again.

But if you are taking prescription estrogen—let's say, to relieve menopausal symptoms—it keeps telling your uterus to build up the uterine lining (with blood), but never to shed it. That's dangerous and has been linked to endometrial cancer, which is cancer of the lining of the uterus.[15] However, when we add progesterone, it signals to the body to shed the lining to avoid that buildup of blood. That is why, whenever a physician prescribes estrogen, they will always also prescribe progesterone. The one exception to this would be if you have had a hysterectomy. If you don't have a uterus, you obviously no longer have to worry about an overly thick uterine lining!

There are different ways to prescribe progesterone. Usually it's given as pills, but the scheduling can be different depending on your health-care provider. You can take estrogen for a few weeks and then add progesterone for a week every month or every few months. But that will likely lead to uterine bleeding—your period. Alternatively, you can take both estrogen and progesterone every day and avoid the bleeding altogether. Different medical providers prefer different systems, but they all work the same way. Many women are thrilled not to have a period monthly, and love to be on continuous progesterone!

LOCAL HORMONES, OR
HORMONES WITH A PAINTBRUSH

I'm about to make a very significant point about the difference between "systemic" hormones (that are meant to support your entire body) and "local" hormones (that are meant only to affect the part of the body to which they are applied). Please make sure you take the time to understand this point because it will have a dramatic impact on your treatment and your understanding of hormones.

All the hormone treatments I've described until this point in this chapter are "systemic." Regardless of whether they are taken by patch, pill, insertion, or ointment, they are developed in dosages and strengths that are intended to circulate throughout your body and help get that hormone everywhere necessary to you. That's an important distinction and one that women often overlook. A patient will say, "My doctor said I can't use hormones," when what their doctor meant was that they couldn't use hormones that circulate throughout the body. Oftentimes when we suggest the patient go back to the physician and ask about local hormones, they get a radically different answer. The hormone treatments I'm about to outline now are all "local" and are meant to affect *only* the vulva and vagina, not to circulate throughout the rest of your body.

Creams, Ointments, and Potions for Vaginal Atrophy

If your vagina hurts and the tissue in the vagina is not healthy and plump as it should be, this is oftentimes a result of your hormones being off balance. Since your vulva and vagina are extraordinarily sensitive to hormonal shifts, they are often the first place where hormonal insufficiencies are felt. This is typically a common problem for postmenopausal women, but younger women who have been on hormonal birth control of any sort, or some women after pregnancy, childbirth, and nursing can have the same problem. Here is a list of hormonal products that may help and explanations as to what differentiates them. If you are thinking that one of these might be right for you, you should speak to your health-care provider.

Topical estrogen. Estrogen cream that you use in the vagina and on the vulva is the gold standard. Usually within two or three weeks of using the cream on the outside and inside of your vagina, you will see a significant difference. It should make the skin healthier and stronger, pinker and plumper. However, there are some common misconceptions that women have about using estrogen in their vagina. Often, they don't understand the difference between topical, or local, estrogen and systemic estrogen. There are a good number of reasons a woman may not want to use a systemic estrogen, although this, too, often stems from misunderstanding, common misconceptions, and bad media coverage. Although systemic estrogen can be very helpful to many women for their vagina, libido, brain, bones, skin, hair, and heart, women who have a history of family cancer may be advised not to use it. I have outlined the issues more extensively on page 129. However, whatever you might decide about systemic estrogen, it is really important to understand that topical estrogen is another thing entirely. It is local and meant only to get into the specific tissue of your vagina. Even though there may be health-care providers who discourage specific women from using regular estrogen systemically, most are fine with women using it locally. Again, this should be something you can discuss at your next medical appointment.

One problem that seems to crop up again and again with these creams is that they can be irritating and messy to use; additionally, you do have to use them regularly to get the results you want. If you are young and trying to heal damage to your vaginal tissue that was the result of pregnancy, birth, nursing, or using birth control, you may use them for a while and then no longer need them. And so it's not such a big deal. But if you are heading into menopause or are in menopause and you need these creams, it will be an ongoing project. Most commonly, these drugs are prescribed to be used more frequently for a few weeks and then applied only two or three times a week. (The only real alternative to these drugs are new lasers that have been developed to treat the same concerns. You guessed it, for more information on those, go to Chapter 13.) In the meantime, the most common topical estrogen products are:

- Estrace and Premarin are creams that are rubbed in the vagina and around the vulvar area. Premarin is made from equine urine, and although it is the least expensive, it is also not bioidentical (see page 136 for a deeper dive into this issue), and as a result, we don't usually prescribe it to patients.
- Vagifem and Invexxy are suppositories that are inserted into the vagina at night and then melt. Vagifem uses an applicator, whereas Invexxy does not, and they are in formulas that melt

differently. You'll have to try them to see which one works best for you.

- Estring is a ring that is inserted into the vagina; it stays there for three months and slowly releases local estrogen.

Any of these product works extremely well. You just have to be committed to maintain the regimen on an ongoing basis.

Alternatives to Estrogen Creams

In the past few years, a number of alternative therapies have been put on the market, and knowing that they are available can be very helpful when you speak to your gynecologist.

- Intrarosa. This is not an estrogen product. It is another hormone, DHEA, which I described earlier and which your body naturally converts into androgens and estrogens, although we are not precisely clear why. After menopause, because your estrogen drops so significantly, DHEA becomes a more important contributor to your sex hormones. The DHEA in Intrarosa is derived from plants and has similar results to Vagifem, but is often not quite as effective. It is also a cream that needs to be used a few times a week.
- Hyaluronic acid is a clear substance that is naturally produced by your body; its main purpose is to help you hold water in your tissues so that your body stays well lubricated and moist. You'll often find it in face creams or moisturizers. It's a great product, but it's not a hormone, so I talk more about it in Chapter 12, where I discuss pain treatments.

Oxytocin

Oxytocin, commonly known as the "love hormone," acts as a neurotransmitter in the brain.[16] It's associated with a mother's attachment to an infant, to milk release in a nursing mother, and to affectionate social interaction. Studies show that when people hug or kiss a loved one, oxytocin levels rise. We know that the hormone is greatly stimulated during sex, birth, and breastfeeding, and studies show that mothers who have higher levels of oxytocin bond more with their babies; in addition, numerous studies show that there is a correlation between oxytocin and our ability to be empathetic.[17] And some studies suggest that if someone is being touched, their oxytocin level rises and, as a result, they feel pain to a lesser degree.[18] When it comes to sex, women talk about feeling a bit "more" when they take oxytocin. It's not universal, but some women experience the frustrating feeling of not "feeling" touch (to their skin, to their lips, or even to their vulva) the way that they used to or want to, and oxytocin can sometimes help with that feeling. So, you might want to consider using oxytocin if you want to "feel more" during sex, if you feel distracted or distant, or if you think your body may have lost some sensitivity.

Oxytocin is not a widely prescribed drug. You may have heard of Pitocin, which is an oxytocin injection used to cause uterine contractions during labor and after delivery, but beyond that, it is not generally used medically. The nasal sprays sold over the counter to "increase trust" contain a tiny amount of oxytocin, but if you want to take it as a sexual aid, it will be a nasal spray or taken sublingually, as a lozenge that you let dissolve under your tongue. There are no standard dosages yet, and side effects can be subtle to nonexistent. You'll need a prescription from a doctor, who will probably have it made by a compounding pharmacy (see page 136).

If you are interested in pursuing oxytocin, find a medical provider who is comfortable prescribing it, or a reputable compounding pharmacy in your area, and go in and speak to the pharmacist who can direct you appropriately. Again, be aware that patients who find oxytocin helpful say it makes a subtle change, not a huge one. It will not give you the whopping points that testosterone, say, might. But as we know, every point counts, and this might give you a few more.

"MY LIBIDO WALKED OFF!": BETTY'S STORY

Betty is a seventy-one-year-old retired clinical social worker who takes long bike rides every weekend. She also travels extensively and is an avid bird-watcher. She is funny and warm; I fell in love with her the first time she came in. Having a great sex life was always part of her marriage of forty-seven years. But a few years ago, toward her late sixties, she told me, "My libido just got up and walked off around the corner. It went away, and it didn't seem like it was ever coming back!"

Betty missed wanting sex with her husband, and he missed being wanted. "We always had a very good sex life," she said. "It was always quite fun, and an integral part of our marriage." But her dwindling desire, coupled with his dwindling ability to have an erection, was a disaster. When I saw Betty, she confessed, "We were just bewildered, wondering what we could do."

After a few sessions, we started Betty on a daily application of testosterone. It took a few months working with Betty to find the levels that were high enough for her to feel an improvement. Once her libido perked up, we also recommended she start using a vibrator. We thought it would help her with her orgasms as well. "I felt very self-conscious," Betty said. "Even though I had used vibrators off and on in the past, they were ineffective, and I wasn't quite sure how to incorporate this to the fullest." But she and her husband worked on it together and incorporated it into their lovemaking. "My libido isn't exactly what it was when I was a young person," Betty said, "but using the testosterone cream has created a great deal of interest in sex, even fantasies, whereas before they were nonexistent." Most important, Betty told me, "I don't approach sexual activity as something to get over with anymore."

And then Betty gave a perfect example of how menopause comes with life and hormone changes, and why it's so important to address both. "Revitalizing sex has given me an enthusiasm for my whole life," she said. "It helps me appreciate and treasure my husband so much more. If there were no fun to look forward to, oh my God, I would throw him out of the house!" Instead, she said, they do fun things together like bicycle riding, playing bridge, and taking trips whenever they can afford it. "We have a good time," Betty told me. "I look forward to playing with him, outside and inside the house! And lovemaking? I thought it was dead and gone. It's so refreshing to know that it's not."

A WORD ABOUT BIOIDENTICAL HORMONES AND COMPOUNDING PHARMACIES

Whether we are prescribing pills, topical creams or pellets, we always strongly encourage patients to use products that are "bioidentical." Bioidentical hormones are products in which the chemical makeup of the hormones exactly matches the chemical makeup of the same hormones in your body. There is a great deal of misleading information out there on what *bioidentical* means. Let's clear this up right now.

> "Bioidentical hormones" does not mean that the hormones are "organic."
> "Bioidentical hormones" does not mean that the hormones are "natural."
> "Bioidentical hormones" does not mean that the hormones are "not really hormones."

It's important to understand that these products are usually manmade and created in a laboratory, *but the molecular components are exactly the same as (identical to) the hormones in your body*. If you test your blood for estrogen or testosterone, the bioidentical versions that were compounded in a laboratory should not be discernible from the same compounds created in your body.

Now, I'm guessing you are asking the same question I first asked when I started hearing about bioidentical hormones. Why in hell would any pharmaceutical company make hormones for you that don't exactly match what your body creates? And the answer is really simple: Products that match your biology can't be patented. Think about it: Bioidentical hormones cannot be patented, the same way you can't patent water, unless you add some flavoring to it. You can't patent estrogen unless there is something different about *your* estrogen. So, drug companies are incentivized to alter the chemical compound because then they can patent the product. As a result, these manufacturers sometimes suggest that the difference in their hormonal compound is an improvement. We haven't found that to be the case.

In recent years, that trend has changed. Since bioidentical hormones are often preferred, either because women feel safer with them or because they are likely to have fewer side effects, drug companies have looked for new ways to patent and market bioidentical hormones. The way that they have done this is by developing better or unique "delivery" systems. That is, since they can't patent the product itself, they try to come up with an easier or more effective way for the hormone to be delivered. That can be by developing a specific cream or spray, or patch or pellet, which contains the hormone. You, the patient, have been the beneficiary because now, the most commonly used hormones are all available, by prescription, in FDA-approved bioidentical formulations!

Here's another common misconception. Often people assume that anything made in a "compounding" pharmacy is bioidentical. But that is not true. Compounding pharmacies are simply pharmacies that make medications on the premises. They often make drugs to order for specific problems or specific doctors. Compounding pharmacies can make bioidentical or nonbioidentical hormones. It's all in what the doctor orders.

Sometimes patients gravitate toward compounding pharmacies because they assume that if the medicine (or hormone) is being mixed specifically for them, it must be safer or "better for them." That is not necessarily the case. Products bought from FDA-approved companies have rigorous safety standards and often are made by machines, and, as such, are not as subject to human error. For that reason, where possible, we try to use bioidentical products that are prepackaged for commercial use and not compounded by a compounding pharmacy. However, compounding pharmacies can often be a good friend for us. When we are using a medication that is not available in a pre-prepared product, we will have it compounded by a compounding pharmacy. And that can be extremely helpful. Also, sometimes compounding pharmacies can make products less expensively than can the manufacturer of a branded product on the market.

So, there you have it. A simple, introductory primer on hormones. But don't let the simplicity fool you. Hormones can be one of the most important ways for you to get added points for your sex life. You will need a trusted medical team to access them, but most likely it will be worth your while if your body isn't making the right amounts of the hormones you need.

CHAPTER 11

DRUGS THAT HELP, DRUGS THAT HURT

> *+/– 50 points*
> *Addressing:*
> *Primary: Pain, Arousal, Desire, Orgasm*

This chapter will give you the scoop on medications on the market today that may be able to help gain you some much-needed points. It will also help you identify those products that you may be currently using that could be taking away points from your sex life. I'll also make some suggestions on how you might want to manage those drugs to get some of those points back in your life. In nearly every case, you will need to discuss these medications further with your health-care practitioner (HCP), both because these medications require a prescription and because your HCP will understand your unique or individualized concerns. My goal here is to make you an educated patient so that you can advocate for yourself to get those much-needed points.

The first drug to be approved for women's sexual health by the FDA was in 2015.[1] That's twenty years after Caverject, the first drug for men's sexual health, was introduced[2] (and seventeen years after Viagra[3]). There are many possible answers to the question of why developments in women's sexual health have lagged so far behind: our unsupported belief that women's sexual issues are all "psychological"; the reality that, in general, women's health studies and treatments lag behind men's;[4] and perhaps most important, our society's ambivalence about women's sexuality. No matter. We have seen a shift in the last few years and there are some drugs on the market that might prove helpful.

I'm always amused when I see an advertisement or a headline that talks about "the female Viagra." Viagra actually will bring a woman's blood into her clitoral and vaginal area in the same way that it brings blood into a man's penis. But usually when people say "the female Viagra," they are looking for a pill that will make sex "better" for women. But what exactly is "better"? Better can be helping women "want" to have sex (desire), get turned on easier (arousal), or even orgasm with less effort. There is no way Viagra can, or even should theoretically, help with those things.

If a guy has a low libido, or can't have an orgasm, chances are Viagra will do nothing. These men need additional medical or psychological intervention. The same applies to women. But we are lucky that there are a few drugs out there that can be helpful for specific problems.

THE DRUGS AND TREATMENTS THAT CAN HELP

Here are some drugs and treatments you should consider if you are having specific sexual issues. They might help gain you a whole bunch of points!

Wellbutrin (Bupropion)

An antidepressant approved in 1985, Wellbutrin is often still prescribed today for depression. Although it is not as popular as it once was because it is not effective for anxiety, it is, however, one of the most powerful pro-orgasm tools we have. It's a dopamine agonist, which means that it helps your body access dopamine, the pleasure hormone deep in the brain's reward zone.[5] At our center, we have found that it works best for women who used to have orgasms but now are having difficulty having them, or for women whose orgasms have gotten weaker; Wellbutrin often restores their old orgasmic capacity with minimal side effects. (Unfortunately, we haven't found it to be successful for women who have never experienced an orgasm.)

Wellbutrin wasn't given FDA approval for orgasm, so if it is prescribed by your doctor for orgasm issues, it would have to be prescribed off-label. It has very limited side effects. A standard dose when used for depression is 300 mg daily. Under the direction of your provider, you can start with a dose of 150 mg daily for a few weeks and see whether that works. Many of our patients find that works for them. If not, talk to your provider about moving up to 300 mg daily for a few weeks. It really should only take two to four weeks for you to feel a difference. If, after a few months, you feel it works for you, great. If not, taper off and move on. There is no reason to stay on it longer.

One thing to consider before going to your health-care practitioner: Wellbutrin is an antidepressant, not an antianxiety medication. Some patients find it actually makes anxiety worse. We've found this in a handful of patients after prescribing it to hundreds, but it's good to know and keep in mind.

So, if you are in the group of women whose orgasms seems to have taken a hiatus, or who are having trouble that you never used to, Wellbutrin is a great first line of attack!

Addyi (Flibanserin)

In 2015, Addyi became the first drug to be approved by the FDA for female sexual dysfunction and it was aimed at women's desire.[6] An entire book could be written about the dramatic pushback. In the end, Addyi was released with so many caveats that it was nearly impossible for women to access it. Its distribution involved physicians and pharmacists taking a special "test" to be able to prescribe and dispense it. (Imagine the irony of that, since so very few other drugs, including opioids and chemotherapy treatments, require special tests for prescribing physicians.) Finally, when Addyi first came to market at upward of $80 a pill, it was so expensive that most women couldn't afford it.[7] At the time of the writing of this book, the manufacturers have rectified that and it has become much more affordable.

Addyi affects the serotonin receptors; for many women, it helps with desire, meaning that, to some degree, it can help restore a woman's natural interest in sex. It is a daily pill and you would need to take it for four to eight weeks to determine whether it is working or not. A completely nonscientific assessment of the efficacy in our patients puts it at about 50 percent. No, it does not make them wake up one morning and start right-swiping on Tinder, nor does it have them running out to meet their partner at lunch for a quickie. What it does seem to do for our patients is make it easier to say yes, either by quieting the part of the brain that usually gives a thumbs-down, or by stimulating the part that thinks, "Wouldn't it be lovely?"

It's important to have realistic expectations if you are going to give the drug a try. Some women hope for and expect immediate lust. But Addyi works subtly and responsively; it doesn't overwhelm you with crazy desire. It just bumps up your interest level a notch or two. Our goal at the center is always to make a patient feel like herself, just a more interested version.

One of the drawbacks of this drug is that it has to be taken every day, and side effects include tiredness, and for some people, dizziness. But it is intended to be taken at night and many women find it helps them fall asleep. If you want to want to have sex, but feel that it's a constant struggle, this might give you some of the points you may be missing and you should consider speaking to your gynecologist or primary care physician about trying Addyi.

Vyleesi (Bremelanotide)

Approved by the FDA in June 2019,[8] Vyleesi is meant to treat problems with desire. However, it is not a pill; it is a self-administered injection that a woman uses when she is about to have sex. Before you panic at the idea of a shot, just know that most patients say it doesn't hurt. It's given to you in an "auto-injector" that is prefilled and pops in your skin with almost no pain.

At our clinic, we don't have extensive experience with the drug yet, but we were involved in some of the early trials. Here's the thing: the drug may work better for arousal than desire, or it may affect both. A refresher: Desire is wanting to have sex, whereas arousal defines your ability to get turned on. A woman needs to have a certain amount of desire already to be willing to use the shot, right? But if we look at newer models of desire, those that talk about needing to get turned on (aroused) before they can access their desire, this drug might hit the mark perfectly. If you find this confusing, do a quick review of Chapters 5 and 7.

Vyleesi also works in the brain. In that way, it is similar to Wellbutrin and Addyi. It promotes something called the "melanocortin 4 receptor," which involves activating internal pathways in the brain that are generally activated during the body's normal sexual response. The specific mechanism whereby Vyleesi improves desire in women is not clear, but it seems to work.

Vyleesi does have a slightly more severe side-effect profile than Addyi. About 40 percent of the women who use it say that it made them quite nauseated the first or second time they tried it. But generally speaking, after that, the nausea problem seems to resolve. You can speak to your physician about prescribing an antinausea medicine for the first few times you try it.

Also, Vyleesi can raise blood pressure by a few points, so women with uncontrolled hypertension shouldn't be using this drug. Once you have seen a physician and your blood pressure is okay, you should be good to go. (Note that at the time of the writing of this book, Vyleesi's manufacturer is trying to make the first few doses either free or very inexpensive, to keep the costs manageable and allow women to try it themselves.)

PRP Injections

PRP, which stands for "platelet-rich plasma," is a procedure that aims to make women's orgasms easier to have or stronger. It is based on other treatments that have used platelet-rich plasma for treatment of injuries.[9]

Platelets are the clotting cells in our blood, but they also have the potential to enhance the healing of muscle, tendon, ligaments, and joints. That is why PRP has been used to help in the healing of sprains, breaks, or other muscle or ligament problems.[10] In the procedure, the patient's blood is taken from their arm, spun down to extract the PRP, and then those platelets are reinjected into the person.

In recent years, physicians started experimenting with injecting PRP into the clitoris and vaginal canal; women who received the treatment have reported that it helps with both orgasms (by making the clitoris more sensitive), and urinary incontinence (accidental leakage while laughing, coughing, or exercising). Unfortunately there are no good studies supporting this claim; however, we have heard from numerous women that it has helped them, and we are not ones to discount anecdotal evidence. Sometimes, it takes so long to get good research on a procedure that we are willing to try it as long as we are convinced that it isn't harmful in any way.

I know the idea of an injection into the clitoris and the vagina seems extremely unpleasant (that was my first reaction!). But patients report very limited discomfort with the procedure. Lidocaine is used topically to numb the area before the first injection (near, but not into, the clitoris). This injection then completely numbs the second injection of the actual PRP. Ironically, most patients find that the blood draw from their arm, which is done to get the blood for the shot, is the most uncomfortable part of the procedure.

The developers claim that there are currently thirteen countries, including the United Kingdom, South Africa, and Brazil, which have centers that perform the procedure and that there have been no significant side effects reported in any of the countries where this is performed. The only potential side effects that we have seen include temporary minimal vaginal blood spotting, hypersensitivity, or excessive orgasms. A number of yeast infections and urinary tract infections have been reported, but we haven't actually seen them ourselves. None of these problems are good, but since these issues are rarely reported and all are manageable, we believe that women can make their own decision regarding trying PRP. The medical practitioners who pioneered this treatment claim that the procedure works about 80 percent of the time.[11] That has not been our experience. We feel that it is effective for urinary incontinence about 80 percent of the time and for help with orgasm about 60 percent, but that is just a rough estimate of our very limited experience.

One note of caution: since this procedure is not accredited by the FDA or any other medical body, and since it is often performed by nonmedical spas or cosmetic establishments, you might want to consider finding a medical office that performs it, as well as making sure you do due diligence and significant research on a provider before you turn over your clitoris and vagina to them.

CREAMS, OINTMENTS, AND POTIONS FOR VAGINAL ATROPHY

If your vagina hurts and the tissue in the vagina is not healthy and plump as it should be, there are many options for treating the problem. This is typically a common problem for postmenopausal women, but younger women who have been on hormonal birth control of any sort, or some women postpregnancy, childbirth, and nursing can have the same problem. I covered some of these in the previous chapter, but they bear repeating here. Here is a list of products that may help and explanations as to what differentiates them. If you are thinking that one of these might be right for you, I encourage you to speak to your health-care provider.

Topical Estrogen

Honestly, estrogen cream that you use in the vagina and on the vulva is the gold standard because it works best. Usually within a week or two of using the cream on the outside and inside of the vagina, you will see a significant difference. It should make the skin healthier and stronger, pinker and plumper. I outlined the issues regarding hormone creams extensively in Chapter 10; you can reread that chapter to educate yourself and then consult with your medical care provider.

Nonestrogen Therapies

In the past few years, a number of alternative therapies have been put on the market, and though they may not work quite as well as the estrogen products, they can also be incredibly effective:

- Osphena is a SERM (selective estrogen receptor modulator), not an estrogen, and it results in your body producing a product which mimics the benefits of estrogen in the vagina. It is a daily pill rather than a cream, but your health-care practitioner might find it on par with estrogen creams in terms of acceptability.
- Intrarosa. This is not an estrogen product. It is another hormone, DHEA, which your body naturally converts into androgens and estrogens, although we are not precisely clear why. Because your estrogen drops so significantly after menopause, DHEA becomes a more important contributor to your sex hormones. DHEA in Intrarosa is derived from plants and has similar results to Vagifem (page 132) but is often not quite as effective. It is also a cream that needs to be used a few times a week.

The more you are educated on available options, the better armed you will be to have a helpful discussion with your health-care provider. And that, in the end, is the goal. You want more points. You need to know how you can access them.

WHAT ABOUT MARIJUANA?

I have limited clinical experience with marijuana, because it's not legal in New York at the time of this writing. We are only now considering prescribing it to our vulvodynia patients, as it has been approved for chronic pain. But many of my patients who struggle with low desire or ability to become aroused have told me that it heightens their ability to become aroused and also makes their orgasms better. That makes sense, because marijuana works on neurotransmitters in the brain that influence pleasure, memory, thinking, and sensory and time perception. It slows inhibitions. We are not clear how it works, but it either raises the pleasure sensations or dulls the mechanism that stops women from having orgasms.

In her book *Come As You Are*, Emily Nagoski describes women's sexual response in terms of the "gas" and the "brakes," with some elements spurring women on to more arousal and other elements inhibiting or stopping women from getting turned on. It would appear that marijuana potentially acts on both aspects.

In my patients' experience, it doesn't seem to make a significant difference if they smoke, vape, or ingest the drug and I haven't had any patients complain about getting pulled into more extensive drug use because of their marijuana use. But obviously, like any nonmonitored drug, it should be approached with a healthy dose of caution and thought. I hope that, over time, it becomes more available to the medical community because I think there are women who would greatly benefit from marijuana but who hesitate to try it because it is currently illegal in many states, or legal only for very specific indications.

THE (POTENTIALLY) PROBLEM DRUGS: BIRTH CONTROL PILLS, IMPLANTS, ANTIANDROGENS, AND ANXIETY MEDICATIONS

Any number of products or drugs that you may already be using or are considering using could be taking away points from your sex life. But by far, the two culprits that we see on a regular basis in our practice are antidepressants/antianxiety medications and hormonal birth control. Here's a really important thing to remember, though. Even if you know that a drug that you are considering using may negatively impact points, taking some away from some people, it does not necessarily mean that it will *do that for you.*

Remember, you are not a statistic. You are an individual. When you are trying to balance between how much you think a medication will be helpful and potential side effects, it may make sense to give the drug a trial run before you decide it is having a negative effect.

The problem comes in when medical professionals don't tell patients about potential negative side effects, either because they don't have time, they think the side effects are unlikely to be an issue, or don't want patients to obsess or worry needlessly. But we have to be honest with patients, because they are the ones who need to make the decision about whether they can live with potential side effects. And when we don't share potential side effects with patients, we often run into trouble.

Nancy came in complaining of severe dryness and pain in her vulva and vagina. She was getting cuts and tears in her vagina every time she had sex. She was thirty-two, too young for typical menopausal symptoms, and yet her vagina looked like a sixty-year-old's. When we told her that her hormonal birth control was probably the culprit, she got extremely pissed off. "I knew it!" she yelled. "This whole mess started about a year after I started on birth control pills. I told my gynecologist, and she kept insisting that pain was not a side effect of that kind of pill." Lo and behold, when we took her off her birth control pills, gave her some hormonal creams to help, and recommended an IUD, within four months her vagina had healed and looked appropriate for a thirty-two-year-old.

The same thing happened to me in 1990, when I was prescribed a low dose of Prozac for anxiety a few years after it came on the market. A couple of weeks after starting, I was elated by the emotional effects. *This must be what normal people feel like*, I thought. *I'm not worrying and rehashing things in my head all the time.*

However, sometime around then, I stopped being able to have orgasms. The doctor who had prescribed the drug failed to mention to me that anorgasmia was a potential side effect, and honestly, it didn't even occur to me. Prozac was new on the market; it was the first SSRI out there, and I had no idea it could affect orgasms. I went into a tail-spin, and I fell into a classic therapist trap: My first thought was that this must be psychological. I started to think that, subconsciously, I was harboring animosity toward my husband, or that something was terribly wrong with the relationship that was making it impossible for me to orgasm.

A few months later, on a visit with the same doctor, I happened to mention the problem, thinking it was a separate issue. He informed me that anorgasmia was a classic side effect of that class of drugs. Who knew? He could have saved me months of angst, as well as countless midnight heart-to-heart talks with my poor exhausted husband.

The bottom line is that most drugs have potential side effects, but "potential" means exactly that. That there may be problem, but not necessarily. Ask your doctor and educate yourself, but don't avoid those drugs altogether. I often tell patients to try a drug for three to six months, then, at the end of that period, to make an educated decision. By that time, they will know how much help the drug provided, and will also know whether they experienced any side effects.

Hormonal Birth Control

Whether you are using Depo-Provera, patches, or pills, hormones in birth control are systemic—which means that they are intended to affect your hormones throughout your body. Hormonal birth control methods are incredibly effective and often women find they can connect more to their sex drive once they are no longer worried about getting pregnant. But many women also experience negative effects that hinder their sex drive. Many patients tell me, "I feel like I have a slipcover on my body."

Here's how the hormones in your body usually work: As your period and the bleeding ends, FSH (follicle-stimulating hormone) and LH (luteinizing hormone) rise, signaling that the oocyte (egg) is ready to be ejected from the ovary. Meanwhile, estradiol, one form of estrogen, is starting to climb as well. A few days later, FSH and LH spike, and this triggers the release of a mature oocyte. Levels of progesterone and estrogen rise for the next two weeks and signal the body to prepare the uterine lining for implantation of an embryo. If no implantation occurs, both estrogen and progesterone levels drop sharply, triggering your next period. If fertilization and implantation do occur, your estrogen and progesterone stay high, in the best of cases, throughout pregnancy, suppressing the spikes of FSH and LH that drive ovulation.

So now, think about it. If you wanted to stop the rise of FSH and LH to stop an egg from being ejected into a fallopian tube and from there into your uterus, you would raise the progesterone and estrogen and that should do the trick. That's exactly what birth control pills do. They come in many formulations, some with more progesterone and some with more estrogen, but in every case, they are intended to raise progesterone and estrogen to stop the spikes of FSH and LH. That's why some people say that the pill is "tricking the body into thinking it's pregnant." That's not entirely true, but it is true enough. The bleeding that happens because you have discontinued the progesterone and estrogen, looks like a period, but it is not really a period because you have actually interrupted the regular ebb and flow of your hormones. Basically, when you are on the pill you are mimicking being pregnant for three weeks and then you have one week of not being pregnant and you bleed as a result.

Now, why are birth control pills problematic for your sex drive? Many forms of hormonal birth control have a secondary effect of lowering your production of natural estrogen as well as testosterone, both of which you really do need to have a sex drive. And to add to the puzzle, most of them also raise your SHBG (sex hormone–binding globulin). As mentioned earlier, SHBGs are proteins in your bloodstream that attach themselves to any testosterone floating around and make them nonusable in your body. So if you have a limited amount of testosterone but a high level of SHBG, your body is not going to have any testosterone to use.

Many, many women use hormonal birth control successfully without it creating secondary problems for their vagina and/or their interest in sex. But some women do find that it affects them negatively and takes away points that they can't afford to lose.

It's important to know that the hundreds of birth control pills out there vary widely in their ingredients. Some have small amounts of estrogen and progesterone; some have larger amounts. Some birth control pills are antiandrogens, specifically designed to shut down your testosterone production. These pills are great for your skin, since testosterone promotes oil and acne. So, think about your sex life. If your vagina has been acting strangely, hurting you or just feeling drier and less sexy, or if you feel that your body isn't responding the way it used to since you started a new form of birth control, think about making a change.

Before you give up on hormonal birth control entirely, have a conversation with your health-care provider. Consider trying the methods with the lowest amount of hormones and the least antitestosterone effects. Your gynecologist, midwife, or nurse practitioner should be able to guide you on this and help you make the right decision. If you do decide to give up on your hormonal birth control, consider using an IUD (intrauterine device).

IUD

The IUD is a small plastic or copper device about the size of a large marble that is placed in your uterus. It makes the uterus less friendly for eggs to implant. There are a bunch of different IUDs on the market now. The classic copper one, available for a decade, unfortunately makes women's periods heavy and long. New iterations, such as Mirena and Skyla, aren't technically free of hormones because they include some progesterone to stop the uterine bleeding, but, it's important to understand that the quantity of hormones found in an IUD is tiny. Because it is very limited, it is considered "local"—that is, it only affects the uterus to limit bleeding, and should not affect the entire body. This means that most women do not experience the side effects of hormonal birth control when they switch to an IUD, but some women do have irregular periods or spotting for three to six months when they are first inserted.

SSRIs and SNRIs—Serotonin/Norepinephrine Reuptake Inhibitors

SSRIs (selective serotonin reuptake inhibitors) as well as SNRIs (serotonin-norepinephrine reuptake inhibitors) are ubiquitous now because they have been invaluable in treating anxiety and depression; there is a wide selection of these drugs on the market. Some of the names of SSRIs you may hear are Celexa (citalopram), Lexapro (escitalopram), Prozac (fluoxetine), Luvox (fluvoxamine), Luvox CR (fluvoxamine controlled release), Paxil (paroxetine), and Zoloft (sertraline). SNRIs include Pristiq (desvenlafaxine), Cymbalta (duloxetine), Effexor (venlafaxine), Savella (milnacipran), and Fetzima (levomilnacipran), and the list goes on. Unfortunately, these drugs can make it harder for a guy to ejaculate and for a woman to orgasm. Around 70 percent of men and women will have trouble climaxing with these drugs.[12] But I'll say it again: you may not. And the best way to tell is to try.

These drugs can be incredibly helpful. When we have a patient who suffers from severe anxiety, we encourage her to try one of these medications, because the reality is that if you are a walking bundle of nerves, you are not going to have a great sex life. These medications can be life-changing and you may not even be one of the people who have a resulting problem with orgasm. Once again, this becomes a cost-benefit analysis. If your physician or psychiatrist points out to you that you have anxiety that warrants medication, try the med before you dismiss it out of hand. If it turns out that you are indeed someone who reacts to the medication with trouble having an orgasm, you may have to work around those −20 points.

- First, you have to decide how important having an orgasm is to you. For some people, the normalcy that they experience once they start taking the medication is significantly more important than having an orgasm. And though orgasms are important to a good sex life, you can certainly survive without them.
- You can use stronger stimulation to have an orgasm and this might be a good time to try out vibrators (see Chapter 14), because the reality is that for some people, the stronger, more intense stimulation will make the difference between having an orgasm or not having one.
- Another option is to speak to your prescribing practitioner and discuss taking a "drug holiday." This means that you try to get off the medication for 48 to 74 hours before having sex. The strength of the medication will often lessen for that period of time and for some people it is enough to enable an orgasm.
- Talk with your health-care provider about trying a different prescription. Recently, two drugs, Trintellix and Viibryd, were put on the market with studies that report a lower profile of sexual dysfunction.

What I hear from so many therapists is that one of the most common reasons people stop taking their antianxiety meds is because of the sexual side effects. The reality, though, is that each person is different, and you'll have to figure out how important those points are for you or whether you can find a medication that doesn't cause that side effect in you. (And note that drug companies are working hard to come up with a formula that doesn't interfere with orgasm.)

Drugs can be extremely helpful in getting points in every one of the four quadrants when you are struggling. They also might be the culprit when new issues arise. Here are the most important takeaways as you think about your current or potential medicine chest:

- You are a person, not a statistic. Just because a percentage of people have certain side effects, does not mean you will. If you feel like a medication could be helpful, you owe it to yourself to try it and see how many points you can gain. You can then make an educated decision.
- Your sex life, like most of your life, is subject to a cost-benefit analysis. Drugs that help in one area might be a problem in another, and that's okay. But only you can make the decision how to balance those. Not your friend, the media, or a health-care provider.
- Medications are usually not "all or nothing." They can be dosed, timed, and adjusted if you have a caring provider who will take the time to listen to your concerns and work with you to find what works best.
- In every situation, the more armed you are with information, the more effective an advocate you can be for yourself. And knowing what drugs and procedures are available to help with each quadrant should make the process of finding help much easier.

CHAPTER 12

THE "NO PAIN" CAMPAIGN

> +80 points
> Addressing:
> Primary: Pain
> Secondary: Desire, Arousal, Orgasm

W hether you have vaginismus, vulvar-vestibulodynia, or genitourinary symptoms of menopause, you need to understand how often contributing factors can overlap. You might have a few different things that are contributing to the pain and as a result, treatments also overlap. This chapter covers some of the most common and central treatment options for painful sex, but I want you to keep in mind that when you are looking to resolve vaginal pain, you will likely need to use a combination of treatments. There probably won't be a single solution.

Before you do anything else, if you are having painful sex, make an appointment to see your health-care practitioner or gynecologist. There are some very basic, obvious things that your primary health-care provider can address, and there are also some more serious conditions that they will likely rule out. It's important to do that before embarking on the journey to find a treatment for your pain. This book is not going to address infections and vaginitis, or the conditions that may cause deep pain and heavy bleeding. Those conditions (endometriosis, fibrosis, and ovarian cysts) are not generally associated specifically with sex; they cause more generalized pain and are usually detected by gynecologists or a primary health-care provider. They can also screen you for IC (interstitial cystitis), which is a bladder condition that you may want to address along with the pelvic pain.

This chapter is going to outline the basics of the most common treatments for pain. Some of these, you might be able to handle on your own. For others, there is no question that you will need medical/professional support or prescriptions; but even in those cases, if you read through these treatment protocols, you will be better able to understand the treatments, appreciate how the subtle differences may affect your situation, and better advocate for yourself. And that's half the battle.

STRETCHING THOSE TIGHT MUSCLES

Using dilators is a central part of the treatment for many, if not all, of the problems I've outlined. Why? Because if the problem is tight muscles, you will need to teach those muscles to relax and stretch more easily. And here's the catch: even if the problem did not start from tight muscles, very often those muscles have reacted to other types of pelvic pain by tightening up. So, even if you fix the other problems, the muscles have to be restretched and learn to relax. For example, a menopausal woman who has a lot of vaginal atrophy (dry, thin, papery vaginal tissue) might be given a topical estrogen cream to "fix" the tissue. But once the tissue is fixed, very often there is residual pain because she's learned to tighten up those muscles in response to the pain. If no one addresses the tight muscles, she's likely to decide that the estrogen "didn't work" and stop using it. And then, she's actually back to square one. In all of these cases, dilators are a central way to do train the muscles to relax and stretch.

Vaginal dilator is a fancy name for a cylinder. Dilators come in varying widths (circumferences) that you introduce into your vaginal canal for short periods of time and keep increasing in size. The goal is to slowly train your vaginal muscles to relax around them.

If you are someone who has had intercourse in the past with little to no problem, it is likely that you can buy dilators and use them on your own to solve the problem. If you are someone who has not been able to insert anything into your vagina, or you have always had pain and fear when you insert something, it's more likely that you may need help with vaginal dilation. Either way, it's important for you to understand what's involved and how vaginal dilation works.

There are many types of vaginal dilators on the market, and if you Google "vaginal dilators," you will find a whole slew. Here's a short guide to help you understand the difference between them and help you choose the ones that might be right for you. There is no "best dilator"; there just may be personal preferences and consideration of how you plan on using them. Do not assume because a dilator is more expensive, it is "better." As you look at dilators for potential purchase, see what makes you feel happiest and most comfortable. Some people love to have bright colors; some like clean white plastic. In the end, you are going to be spending quite a bit of time with your dilators, so take some care in thinking about how they make you feel.

Things to Consider When Buying Dilators

MATERIALS

Dilators are made from plastic, silicone, or glass. This affects how easy they might be to insert, how they feel, and how they look. Often women have strong opinions about this issue.

- **Plastic.** The most commonly used dilators are hard white plastic; they are also the least expensive. The commercially sold ones are hollow; medical grade ones are solid and heftier—and those latter are the kind we like to use in the office. There's no right or wrong here, but we do find that patients have an easier time inserting a dilator that is solid and has a bit of weight to it. We use the hard white dilators from Syracuse Medical for our regular dilation patients who do daily ten minute or so dilation. They are no fuss, no muss, easy to clean, and work well.

- **Silicone.** These dilators are generally colorful and bright, and softer, because, well, they are not hard plastic. They tend to be more expensive than the hard plastic ones; another downside is that they are not quite as rigid. We find that when you are trying to push in a dilator against muscles that are a bit resistant, it is easier with something more rigid that has less bend. However, the softer silicone dilators tend to be better and more comfortable if you are sleeping with your dilator (as with our Botox patients).

- **Glass.** Bet you didn't know there were glass dilators, did you? First, please understand that these dilators are shatterproof; they cannot break in your vagina. (Something told me that you weren't going to read another word until I got that out of the way.) Trust me. You will not end up in the ER with glass splinters! These dilators really tend to be more "specialty" dilators. I would suggest that you have another set of basic dilators and buy these as an add-on, rather than as a regular tool. (Think of a little black dress that you wear all the time, and then a splashy red number that you wear on special occasions.) They are significantly shorter in length than regular dilators and therefore will be more likely to stay in if you try to sleep with them. They are also prettier, and frankly, who doesn't want a sex tool that's prettier? And finally, they are good for holding temperature, so if you like the idea of inserting something warm (because it is cozier for your vagina) or cool (because it dulls the pain for you), then these dilators would be great additions. They are the most expensive and come in the least options of sizes.

SIZE

Size is a critically important issue to consider because in the end, the stretching you're doing is all about increasing in size. Let me be clear, though: we're talking the size of the diameter and circumference (how thick or wide they are). The length is not really important because you are not inserting the whole thing into your vagina.

Gradation between sizes may be the most important element in your decision. You want dilators that don't make a huge jump between one size and the next. The dilators we use (Syracuse Medical) have nine sizes: XS, XS+, S, S+, M, M+, L, L+, and XL. The gradations between them are extremely gradual and manageable for our patients. Some companies make only four to six sizes and, with those, we've found that patients have a difficult time sometimes transitioning from one to the next.

You also want to keep an eye out for the largest size available in a set. In the end, you are dilating to get your vagina to stretch without pain to a smidge larger than your partner's penis (if your partner has a penis). That's because we want you to be able to have intercourse without worrying at all about pain. Some dilator sets only go to large, some go to large-plus. In truth we needed to add an even bigger white plastic dilator to our stock from a totally different source, because a few of our patients had partners with a larger penis and we needed to help them stretch larger than their partner's penis. If you are just starting out in the dilation process, this is probably less of an issue for you. Start with a standard set. At the point where you get to the larger ones and are concerned that your partner's penis might be girthier, just measure the aforesaid penis, and then you can always purchase a larger dilator or a dildo that will help you stretch just a tad bigger.

As noted, you don't need to worry about length. That said, if you intend on sleeping with a dilator in, you'll want to choose a shorter dilator with a lip around the edge, for comfort. Either a silicone or glass dilator will work.

"So now that I've purchased a dilator set, how do I use them, Bat Sheva?"

Well, that depends on many factors. If you buy them online, they may come with instructions, but the concept is the same no matter what dilators you purchase. Here is a straightforward guide:

1. You want to insert the largest one that can go into your vagina without significant discomfort. You will push it in until it feels as though it can't go any further. Now, that first dilator might be uncomfortable and hurt a bit. The whole issue might freak you out and it might burn or pinch a little. Don't push too hard. Three to 4 inches are sticking out, that is FINE. The muscles you are trying to stretch are the ones that go around and grip the penis; you are not trying to lengthen your vagina.

   If you are breathing heavy from pain and feeling like you just can't do it . . . it's too big!! Go to a smaller size. See whether you can find a dilator that you can put in with some gentle breathing and relaxation, and one that feels like it is tight, or burning a tad but it gets better after a minute or two of lying there. That's the right size. There's really no harm at all with starting with the smallest size, if that's easier. Just use it for a day or two and then try moving up. Starting with a smaller size means it will take a bit more time to move up to the size you want. But, hey, you've been living with this condition for a while. An extra week or two won't make a huge difference.

   A couple of things to note: Classically, women with vaginismus have the worst trouble just pushing the dilator through the first set of muscles at the entrance to the vagina because these muscles are the ones that are tightest. Often women will say as soon as they get past that ring of muscles, the vagina feels wide open, soft, and pliable.

   Another thing that women tell us is that they have an indescribable "yicky" feeling when they pull the dilator out. It's not pain, they say, it just feels weird, uncomfortable, and they feel queasy. We're not sure what that's about, but we suspect that the feeling of the muscles tightening up as the dilator pulls out, is just new and unexpected. After a few weeks of dilating, most women tell us they feel that it's so much better.

2. Once you insert the dilator, you want to spend a minimum of ten minutes or so just lying there with the dilator inserted, while you relax. Try watching a TV show or listening to a podcast. You may not be able to use social media or email because it is likely, at least in the beginning, that you will have to hold the dilator in place. Those tight muscles are really happy to squeeze down and expel the dilator if nothing is holding it in place. Once you are able to slide a dilator in without too much pain and relax to a place where it no longer hurts significantly, you then should start moving it, up and down and around (remember you are trying to stretch the muscles around the vagina).

3. At the point when a dilator stays in and you can move it around without too much discomfort, you are ready for the next size. Sometimes, women want to wait until they don't feel the dilator at all, or there is absolutely no pressure or discomfort, before they move up to the next size. That's probably not a good idea. Usually the largest size you are using is uncomfortable when you first put it in, and it often stays that way until your body adjusts to the next size up. Only once you have gotten used to a new larger size, the last one you used (the smaller size) then becomes totally comfortable. That's why we want you to get to a size that's just slightly bigger than whatever you want to insert. That largest dilator might never get 100 percent comfortable, but your partner's penis, a dildo, or a tampon should now be fine.

FAQs/Troubleshooting

"DO I NEED A THERAPIST OR CAN I DO THIS ON MY OWN?"

Some women, once they know how to dilate, can do it on their own. Typically, postchildbirth, menopause, or sudden onset of tight muscles is much more easily self-treated and you can do it on your own.

If that's you, you go girl! But if that isn't you . . . don't panic, it's fine! The women who have never been able to insert anything and have a fear component may have a much harder time of it. But don't give up. You just need someone to help you get started. A pelvic floor physical therapist is a great option for this, or if you are lucky enough to have an ob-gyn who can take significant amounts of time with you, coaching, holding your hand, and breathing, that's good as well.

"I'M JUST SO ANXIOUS ABOUT PUTTING SOMETHING INSIDE!"

If you have a lot of anxiety, then now would be the time to see a psychotherapist who has expertise in this area. And you should see the psychotherapist while you are going through the dilation process. I'd be wary of a therapist who tells you to stop dilating until you are no longer stressed by the idea. In my opinion, that is not helpful. This condition is one that is best approached by actually doing the exercises and working it through at the same time. Think of someone who has a fear of heights. Exposure therapy has them going higher and higher with the appropriate support. If they just talked about the fear of heights, they might be talking for years without actually making progress. Sometimes, women are reassured by therapists that if they talk enough, they will no longer be scared or anxious. That's not our experience. We feel that working on both things together makes all the difference.

In looking for a good therapist to help you through this, try to find someone who is comfortable with body work and somatic therapy (understanding how the body is affected by stress). The most effective therapy to help you through dilating will include deep breathing as well as antianxiety guided-imagery mind/body work to help you relax your mind and body while you introduce the use of dilators. This might also be a time to consider antianxiety medication to help you through the process of dilation. (See Appendix II, page 271, for tips on finding the right therapist.)

"I KNOW MY MUSCLES ARE TIGHT, BUT THERE IS NO WAY IN HELL I WILL BE ABLE TO DILATE. NOW WHAT?"

Maybe the idea of using dilators literally makes you want to vomit or faint. Or you have tried physical therapy and are not making progress. Honestly, if you just want to jump-start the process and solve it faster, consider doing Botox injections with dilation under anesthesia.

I wrote quite a bit about this in Chapter 4, but here is a refresher: A patient is put under conscious sedation for fifteen to twenty minutes, while a physician gently presses on the first ring of tight muscles, allowing them to loosen up and give. If a hymenal ring is still there, it's trimmed, Botox and lidocaine are then injected up and down the whole vagina and the large dilator is then inserted. Voilà. The patient "wakes up" after a few minutes, usually calm and relaxed from the residual anesthesia, and feels no pain at all, because of the lidocaine in the vagina. She sees for herself, that her vagina is fine. It can handle a dilator. All is well with the world. The Botox takes a few days to fully "kick in", but by day 5, the patient can't tighten those muscles and that gives her time to dilate with the extra help of medically relaxed muscles. Within a few months, the Botox wears off, but by then, patients have dilated to the point where they can relax the muscles. We have seen incredibly few situations where the Botox needed to be reinjected.

If you are considering Botox treatment for tight muscles, here are the most important things to consider:

- Botox doesn't solve the problem; it just jump-starts solving the problem.
- You need a health-care practitioner *who uses dilation with the Botox procedure*. We've seen too many women who've had Botox injections and say it didn't work, because their practitioner sent them home after the injection with no dilators and/or didn't show them how to work with dilators after the injection.

- You still need psychological support! Make sure you find a good therapist to work with you.
- It can be a bit of an expensive proposition because medical procedures, especially in the US, are costly.

We have seen women respond really well to this treatment, and the results are often amazing and fast. Sure, it's expensive. Sure, it sounds scary. But the truth is, you may have been living with this condition for a very long time. And I'm guessing it's getting in the way of how you feel about yourself and possibly, as a result, you are avoiding relationships or feeling alienated from your partner. This procedure can be life-changing, and it may be worth saving up for a few months, if you can. Don't let this problem linger. It can be insidious and affect other parts of your life that can be harder, and pricier, to heal in the long run.

"VALIUM FOR MY WHAT???"

When we are working with women to help them relax and stretch their pelvic floor muscles, we will often give them Valium suppositories to insert at night before they go to bed. Yes, it's the same medication that people are given to help relax their brain, but these suppositories melt in the vagina and help to relax those tight muscles. Using them alone, without dilation, probably won't help a lot, but many of our patients find that using them helps make the dilation just that much easier and they get faster results. The suppositories need to be compounded for you by a specialty pharmacy, but see your health-care provider and they should be able to arrange for that to happen.

"I THINK IT MIGHT ACTUALLY NOT BE JUST MY VAGINA."

If you are someone who has sexual pain, but also know that your pelvic region is tight in general, then it's time to make an appointment with a local pelvic floor physical therapist. How do you know whether your pelvis is tight? Well, if you've chronically had bowel or urinary problems, or if you have been told that your hips or quads or glutes are extremely tight. Often, when you tighten up part of that region, other muscles get pulled into the party. You may not realize how much tension you are holding in your butt, or your vagina, but the areas surrounding them might give you telltale clues.

In those cases, going to a pelvic floor physical therapist can be invaluable. They'll give you stretching and loosening exercises, and they might actually get up close and personal to your vaginal and rectal muscles to help with the stretching. Make sure you find someone who is licensed as a pelvic floor therapist and who seems to have good reviews regarding rapport with the patients. This is obviously a sensitive area for physical therapy and it's important that you have someone with whom you are comfortable and who you trust.

TOPICAL MEDICATION FOR HORMONAL IMBALANCES

Another component of pain is vaginal tissue affected by hormones being off balance. When your body experiences a drop in estrogen and testosterone, your vulva, vagina, and all the tissue surrounding it are the first to feel the effect. They can get red, tissue paper thin, and easily irritated. Hormonal birth control, childbirth, and nursing as well as just plain age and menopause can do this. The best solution for this problem is a topical hormonal cream or gel that you use on the vulva and/or the vagina.

The best long-term fix for these problems is a combination of changing or removing the underlying cause of the problem (if that's possible), and then using a cream, ointment, or suppository to put back the hormone that your body is missing. Obviously if you are menopausal, you can't change the underlying problem. But if the pain and low hormones are due to your use of hormonal birth control, you may want to seriously consider changing that.

I encourage you to revisit Chapter 10 on hormones, specifically the descriptions of all the hormonal creams, ointments, and suppositories that can help. The first line-of-defense creams you should consider are estrogen cream, a combination estrogen and testosterone cream, or DHEA cream. Take a look at pages 130–134 and then discuss this issue with your health-care provider. This is one of those times when information is power.

I'm going to repeat something I said in Chapter 10, because it is critical that you understand the difference between systemic and local hormone treatment. The drugs I'm suggesting are all local! That means that these drugs are meant to help just the specific area of application, do not get into the rest of your system, and are therefore less concerning to health-care providers, while they are critical at giving you back the hormones that your vulva and vagina might be missing. Try not to be scared of them; they can be helpful.

Okay, It's Not Actually a Hormone, but Still: Hyaluronic Acid

Hyaluronic acid is a fluid that is naturally part of our body. You see most of it in the eyes and joints (as a matter of fact, to treat dry eyes, it is sometimes injected to help replace natural fluids). There are any number of ways you can use hyaluronic acid to help with the effects of aging and dryness in your vagina, because it is available in both gel form and as pellet suppositories. There are reputable over-the-counter products (Hyalo Gyn or Revaree are two). And if you prefer to work with a medical provider, you can always find a good compounding pharmacy to prepare a formulation for you with a prescription from your provider. It is an alternative to local estrogen, and it will help you regain some of the moisture and suppleness. It is not as effective as an estrogen cream, but if you, or your health-care provider, are not comfortable using an estrogen cream for some reason, it can be a helpful alternative.

It's All About the Base

There are women with incredibly sensitive skin, who can't seem to tolerate many of the creams and ointments that they are prescribed. They find that those burn, itch, or irritate. In those cases, we will have the medications that they need compounded, without perfumes or alcohol, by a specialty pharmacy. Some pharmacies will mix the medication into a base that they know won't irritate the patient and the patients essentially get a customized cream, without the trial and error and without spending a lot of money on creams that they couldn't continue to use. So, check that out with either your health-care practitioner or your local compounding pharmacy, if you are worried that creams and lotions often irritate you.

You may want to speak to your health care practitioner about trying some of these topicals even if they aren't sure that the lack of hormones has contributed to your problem or if they don't "see" a problem. Using topicals for a month is the best way to judge whether they will help. You can absolutely use them while you are dilating or working on other treatments, and within a month, you will be able to tell if they are helping.

Treatment for Overactive Nerves

This is the hardest part of the chapter to write, because if I'm honest, the medical community has not really figured out a great solution for overactive nerves. As a result, the treatments tend to be more trial and error and scattershot. Women can great results, but it often takes a great deal of patience and stubbornness to get help. In every case, you will need a medical professional help to navigate the solutions. Here is a list of products that might help:

- **Nerve pain–specific drugs.** There are oral medications that affect the nerves in your body and make them less sensitive.

Two common ones are Lyrica (pregabalin) and Neurontin (gabapentin); both of these drugs are approved to treat nerve pain, including fibromyalgia and diabetes pain. Neither of these drugs heals the pain, but they often make daily life more manageable. Dosages are different for different drugs, so you'll need to discuss this with your health-care provider.

- **Antidepressants.** Another class of drugs that can be helpful for overactive nerves is tricyclic antidepressants. Elavil (amitriptyline) is used most often for depression at higher doses, but the same mechanism that helps with depression, raising the body's serotonin levels, also seems to change your body's reaction to pain at lower doses. A secondary advantage to the lower dose is that it helps you sleep. These medications are most commonly used orally, taken in pills. But many of us who specialize in this field also use these medications topically. We have them compounded by specialty pharmacies. Gabapentin and Neurontin are often used in creams, and one popular combination cream is ABG cream: amitriptyline, baclofen (a muscle relaxant), and gabapentin. Sometimes lidocaine anesthetic cream or diazepam (a muscle relaxant) is also used in combination with these, as are mixtures including these and the hormonal creams I touched on earlier. If this all seems too complicated or overwhelming for you, take this chapter with you to your health-care practitioner, and see whether they can help with navigating the medications.

- **Capsaicin.** Another prescription medication used to tame those overactive nerve endings is capsaicin, a chile pepper extract with pain-relieving properties. Nope. You don't eat it on your sloppy joe. It's a cream used on the vulva, and honestly, it burns like hell. While we don't know exactly how it works, it's thought to release a chemical that blocks some of the pain signals from sensory nerve fibers to the brain. Women have found that it gives them some relief from their nerve pain, and despite the burning, are willing to use it periodically to keep the pain at bay.

- **Cold level laser.** I talk more about that in Chapter 13 on lasers, but it's worth a brief mention here as well. A cold level laser has been shown in small-scale studies to reduce vulvar pain. Although not many pelvic pain centers have the laser, or know how to use it, it's a great option and you should know about it. It involves painless and short-term treatments, and usually you will know within a month whether it is going to work for you.

LET'S TALK ABOUT SURGERY

I know you don't want to hear this, there is always surgery. A vestibulectomy cuts away the section of the vestibule that has overactive nerves. There are good studies that show 61 to 94 percent improvement or cure after vestibulectomy.[1] It's a major surgery and I won't lie: it's a truly miserable surgery. You have to stay flat on your back for a while, and your mobility is limited for weeks. But, and here's the good news: it usually is successful. So, that means that you may well be pain-free forever after the surgery. And sometimes short-term misery can really be worth it for long-term gain.

A FINAL WORD ON CURING PELVIC PAIN

Samantha came to us after having seen at least five health-care practitioners: three gynecologists, one endometriosis specialist, and one pelvic floor physical therapist. She was aggravated, frustrated, starting to doubt herself and giving up on ever finding a solution. Tiny and ferocious, she started off our relationship by throwing down the gauntlet. "Yeah. No way you're gonna help me," she said. Then, with a big sigh, "I figured, what the hell? I'll try one more time." She really didn't think we'd be able to help, which is always challenging for us, because that means that we needed to gain her trust as well as navigate the presenting issues. The truth is, as I tried to explain to her, some of those practitioners she saw actually gave her good advice: discontinuing her hormonal birth control and using hormonal creams and doing vaginal stretching exercises. The problem was that each gave them to her in isolation and didn't pay attention to the whole picture. And that's critical when you are dealing with pain. She needed to address all three of those issues, possibly in a particular order. Once she understood that, and we got going, she healed quickly and efficiently. And once she trusted us, Samantha turned out to be a model patient, trying the remedies we suggested, reporting back if they didn't work, and barreling ahead with alternatives. After a few months, her pain was almost all gone. Then, we needed to work with her on repairing the damage to the relationship. But that's a story for another chapter.

What we have seen over the years in our practice, is that physicians may give patients only one piece of the puzzle when they are addressing a patient's pain or, even more concerning, they are unwilling to think outside the box. And that just doesn't solve the whole problem. For example, we have seen hundreds of women in their forties and fifties who have been given estrogen cream when they go see their gynecologist because their vagina has atrophied. But their medical practitioners can't imagine why they'd need dilators (which they think of as only for young, newly sexually active patients). In those cases, the muscles have also tightened up and the health care providers didn't address that at all, because they can't imagine that a woman who had perfectly fine intercourse for years, now has tight muscles. Similarly, we've seen young women whose vagina looks menopausal because of their hormonal contraceptives, but their health-care providers never thought to give them estrogen cream because that is for "older women." It's time we stop thinking of women entirely as a category and understand that there might be significant overlap.

I truly meant it when I said that you may need to use a number of treatments to get pain-free. And it's all good. Make sure you find a health-care provider who takes you seriously, understands the complexity, and is willing to work with you in trial and error until you get to a place that makes you happy. You deserve it, and the number of points that you can get by fixing your vulva and vagina are incredibly important and almost irreplaceable.

CHAPTER 13

LASERS
Zap Your Way Out of Pain

> *+30 points*
> *Addressing:*
> *Primary: Pain*
> *Secondary: Desire, Arousal*

Lasers aren't exactly sexy, but I do know that they could turn out to be a good friend when it comes to pelvic pain.

It's not clear when medical lasers began to be used to treat women's vulvar and vaginal issues, and it's important to understand that not all machines we think of as lasers are actually lasers; some just look like or function like lasers. (*Laser* stands for "light amplification by stimulated emission of radiation.") Patients tend to call lasers any device that uses a "beam" of some sort, but the reality is that often what we think of as lasers are machines that use other types of waves, such as radio or sound, to promote healing.

In the past few years, there has been a big proliferation of laser (or laserlike) procedures that actually can help repair the vulva and vagina.[1] Some of them solve problems otherwise not solvable. And some of them just make it much easier to treat issues.

FRACTIONAL CO_2 LASER FOR POSTMENOPAUSAL PAIN

You're perimenopausal or postmenopausal and your vagina hurts when you have intercourse. You may not be able to fully describe the pain. It's weird. You may feel a sharp pain, or a burning, or just plain irritation. This is because the mucosa (what you probably think of as the skin) in the vagina has gotten thin and irritated and tears easily. Because the vagina is so sensitive to hormonal shifts, when your natural level of estrogen drops, your vagina can be the first part of your body to feel the difference.[2]

If you've seen your gynecologist for this, you may have been told that there is no problem—and that is probably because the problem hasn't gotten bad enough to be seen or because the problem is actually tight muscles, not the outside layer mucosa. But if your doctor does see the skin or mucosa in your vagina getting "old" (thinner, or papery, or dry), you have most likely been told to use an estrogen cream to help heal the tissue and mucosa.

As mentioned earlier, using an estrogen cream will totally help the problem and that's great. But if you can't use estrogen because of a history of breast cancer or if you just don't like using daily creams, laser and laserlike treatments are an option—and more and more gynecologists are offering them in their office.[3]

The most popular and widely known lasers for this condition are the fractional CO_2 lasers.[4] You might have heard them called the Mona Lisa Touch, or the Femilift (there are other lasers being used for the same purpose). Here is a simple rundown on how they work:

Using the Mona Lisa Touch as an example, a fractional CO_2 laser is put into your vaginal canal with a vaginal probe. The laser beams target both the surface and deep tissue and stimulate small injuries in the epithelial layer of the vaginal mucosa. Basically, you're damaging the outer layers, which triggers fibroblast activity to stimulate your body to "heal." In doing so, you create new collagen, elastin, and more new blood vessels.

I know it sounds like it would hurt, but it mostly doesn't. A numbing cream is put on the surface during the procedure so that it doesn't hurt. While there is some pain for a few days after the procedure, it is brief and then, voilà, you have new tissue and mucosa developing in the vagina. Since the procedure is safe and virtually painless, women really love it as an option. Usually, you need three treatments; when things start to get irritated again (maybe after a year or two), you can get touch-ups. Currently, the procedure is not covered by insurance, so it can be pretty expensive.

LLLT OR COLD LASER THERAPY FOR CHRONIC PELVIC PAIN

Low-level laser therapy (LLLT), or, as it is sometimes called, cold laser therapy (CLT), uses red and NIR (near infrared) light. Used to treat chronic pain conditions, such as lower back pain, bursitis, and carpal tunnel syndrome, LLLT applies low levels of red and NIR light to an injury or a trigger point. It then penetrates the skin and the tissue so that there will be greater blood flow and less inflammation, and hopefully the tissue will regenerate faster.[5]

It's used the same way for pelvic and vulvar pain. The probe is slowly moved around the surface of the vulva to promote the rejuvenation of the tissue and a lessening of the pain. It's gotten mixed reviews. But one thing's for certain: If, after a few treatments, you don't see an improvement, don't keep going.

The exception to this would be if you have been told that your vulvar pain is neuroproliferative. That is, if your vulvar pain is due to overactive nerve endings and your next option is surgery (see page 44), then a different protocol might be needed for this: cold laser. In that case, the suggested number of treatments is twelve. You would start with six, and if you see an improvement, you would continue to twelve. Not many places are using this protocol, so you may have to do some research to find the right provider.[6]

RADIOFREQUENCY DEVICES

Radiofrequency devices emit electromagnetic waves that generate heat on the tissue. In the past, it has been used for many aesthetic procedures on the face and body and sometimes for fat removal. It has mixed reviews on efficacy but is very safe. More recently, it has been used for urinary incontinence, and seems to be successful with this. It has also been used for vaginal laxity. *Vaginal laxity* is a term that always scares me because I am afraid it is playing on women's fears of getting older and wrinklier.

However, radiofrequency devices are also being touted as a way to "tighten" the vagina and increase sensation for sexual pleasure. There do seem to be some data to back up the claims and if that idea is appealing to you, do some research to see what is out there.[7] There are a whole host of these devices under different names: Protégé Intima, Viveve, ReVive, and Pellevé are a few of the ones out in the US. Again, these procedures are not covered by insurance and can be quite costly, so do your research before you rush in, and keep your expectations fairly modest. These devices can be helpful in gaining you some points, but they likely can't solve the problems all by themselves.

Lasers have turned out to be a real gift when it comes to offering alternative treatments for vaginal issues. And, as you now know, the pain quadrant can significantly impact the others. So, these newer therapies should be appreciated and used whenever it's appropriate. However, sometimes I hear the words "vaginal rejuvenation" in relation to these laser treatments and it makes me cringe!

The treatments I've described in this chapter do, actually, rejuvenate the mucosa inside the vagina. But when I hear women talking about "rejuvenating" their vagina, I am concerned that they are describing something else, something less measurable and more insidious. I think many women somehow think that their vagina gets old, loose, baggy, wrinkled, ugly or just plain useless. Advertisers are quick to use words that bring up those feelings in women because it has been discovered that women will pay anything to be "young," "fresh," and "appealing."

So, let me say this. There is nothing wrong with your vagina, and there is truly nothing better about a younger vagina, except that the mucosa can get dried out when your natural estrogen drops as you age. So, if you are thinking of vaginal rejuvenation as plumping up the mucosa, go for it. But if you think the laser will restore your twenty-year-old vagina, which you believe was more interesting for some reason than your fifty-year-old vagina, maybe talk this through with someone first.

The bottom line is that there's no guarantee that these laser treatments will help more than traditional treatments might, but they are safe and, in some cases, might be very effective. They may help you pick up some extra points in a way that is easy to live with and not overwhelming, so if you have the financial capacity to consider them, they are not at all a bad way to garner some extra points.

CHAPTER 14

VIBRATORS ARE NOT KINKY SEX TOYS; THEY ARE YOUR FRIEND

+60 points
Addressing:
Primary: Arousal, Orgasm
Secondary: Desire

O ften dismissed as kinky sex toys (and there's actually nothing wrong with those), vibrators are some of the most underused tools in women's sexual arsenal. They don't directly help with low desire, but they sure as hell can help with arousal and with orgasm. And they might even help with desire if your lack of desire is actually a result of not getting adequately turned on or not having satisfying orgasms. They help women have orgasms. They help women have more fun with sex. They help women fit sex into a busy, crazy life. They help women say yes to sex because they make it faster and easier. And for women without a partner or with a partner who doesn't have a penis, using the kind of vibrator that goes inside their vagina can feel great.

Vibrators are an easy way to gain yourself a whole bunch of points. They are medication-free, they don't mess with the hormones in your body, and they don't change your physical makeup. They can save time when you are in a rush and allow you to have sex even when you're tired or it's not the most convenient.

Irma was one of my favorite patients. She was eighty-one, definitely in the older demographic of our patients, and the loveliest person. She was a small, white-haired ball of energy who loved to travel and bird-watch. Every time I saw her, it made me smile. Irma hadn't had orgasms in a long time. She didn't even remember the last time she had had one, and she was feeling really sad that her sex life was disappearing. She was in a long-term happy relationship, but she and her husband had somehow let sex slip off the radar.

Our work with Irma was varied and we suggested some medications as well as some practical homework assignments. But a turning point came when I spoke to Irma about incorporating a vibrator into her sex life with her husband. I'll admit, at first, she was really taken aback and a bit resistant. "Really?" she said. "Bat Sheva, you can't teach an old dog new tricks." This made me laugh and I responded that (1) you certainly can teach an old dog new tricks, and (2) she was nothing like an old dog. After some time, she agreed to try the vibrators in our office and I'll never forget the beaming smile on her face when, after she pressed the buzzer for me to come into the exam room, I knocked and entered. "I'm guessing from the look on your face that the vibrator actually worked well for you?" She almost giggled as she told me that not only had she gotten turned on, she'd had an orgasm right there in the exam room.

We then talked a bit about how she might bring this up with her husband. We role-played and discussed some scenarios, but the truth was that she was in a loving, supportive relationship and she figured her husband, who might initially be thrown for a loop, wouldn't be too hard to convince to get with the program. And she was absolutely right.

A few months later, when she came in for a follow-up, she assured me that things were going "splendidly. As a matter of fact, last week, I was miffed because I thought he was spending too much time fussing with our videos from our last trip to Italy. And I was feeling kind of neglected. When he came into the bedroom, he found the vibrator already plugged in and sitting on his pillow waiting for him. He burst out laughing. But he got the message."

Here's the deal. If eighty-one-year-old Irma can figure out how to incorporate vibrators into her sex life, so can you!

Here's a "should I try a vibrator?" quiz (hint: if you say yes to any of these, you should try a vibrator):

- We don't have sex very often because it's such a production. It takes me too long to orgasm.
- I often don't want to have sex because it's so much damn work.
- I never masturbate because it takes so long.
- I'd like to have sex more often if I could figure out a way to do it even when I'm exhausted.
- If my orgasms were stronger, I'd want sex more.

A QUICKIE COURSE ON VIBRATORS

There are more types of vibrators out there than you can imagine. Really. There are big ones, little ones, internal ones, external ones, strong ones, weak ones, soft ones, hard ones, long ones, short ones, vibrators shaped like animals, and vibrators that talk to you. The only thing I haven't seen is a vibrator that tells you the time, but I'm sure they are working on that.

The most important thing to remember is that even though there may be a million "different" vibrators out there, they are all essentially variations on a few themes. So basically, if you are familiar with four to six types of vibrators, then you have all the information you need and can pretty much assess the subtle differences and choose accordingly.

The first distinguishing factor you need to think about is external vs. internal. That is, there are vibrators that are meant to go inside your vagina and others that are meant to be used externally on your clitoris. Let's start by reviewing the latter kind because I think, for the most part, they are used more and are more helpful to more women.

Clitoral (or External) Vibrators

These vibrators are meant to be used externally, directly on your clitoris, and may be shaped like a very thick pen, egg, or microphone. They may be curved, with wide cup handles. They are clearly not meant to be used internally because they are either not long enough and would be hard to reach inside the vagina, or they are too wide and would be painful to insert. These vibrators are best if you want clitoral stimulation (usually for orgasm).

They can be used alone or with your partner, with either you or your partner holding the vibrator. Often these vibrators make it easier to have an orgasm than stimulation from a hand or mouth.

Actually, now would be a good time to repeat an important statistic: Only 30 percent of women have an orgasm from intercourse alone, 70 to 80 percent have an orgasm from a hand or a mouth, and 95 percent can have an orgasm from a vibrator. So, you can see why using an external vibrator might be an attractive option.

External vibrators come in battery-operated or plug-in/chargeable models. The battery-operated ones tend to be smaller and subtler. Some are even fitted to go on the penis. Many women gravitate toward the small battery-operated ones. The important thing to keep in mind is that the plug-in or rechargeable models are significantly stronger, so if one of the reasons you're considering using a vibrator is that you are having trouble having an orgasm, it's taking too long, or they are not strong enough, you should probably buy a plug-in or chargeable one.

There are three things to consider when choosing an external vibrator: strength, appearance, and noise level.

STRENGTH

This is by far the most important factor to consider. Vibrators can vary significantly in terms of the amount of pressure they provide. Every woman is different in the amount of pressure, stimulation, and speed she finds arousing. Generally speaking, younger women prefer lighter or weaker vibrators and older women prefer the stronger ones. However, this is one of those cases where really and truly each woman needs to find out what feels good to her individually.

Most of the external vibrators are on the smaller side and, as a rule, are battery operated. Although battery-operated vibrators can get pretty strong, they are not ever as strong as the plug-in or rechargeable models, and the batteries tend to drain fairly quickly. If you're using a battery-operated vibrator, make sure you have a large supply of whatever batteries your vibrator calls for on hand, and if a vibrator feels "weaker than it used to," it is probably a signal to replace the batteries. You do not want to be in the throes of passion, about to orgasm, and have your vibrator conk out on you. It's not pleasant.

If you are having trouble with orgasms, I would highly recommend that you immediately go to a stronger vibrator. Choose a plug-in or chargeable model. Some women (young or old) just need the repetitive, strong stimulation that a vibrator can give and a strong, plug-in model is the best way to achieve this.

APPEARANCE

External vibrators can be cute, funky looking, or subtle. They also can be "in your face" and quite noticeable, so take your time picking one out. You'll have to live with it for a while.

The plug-in and chargeable models tend to be bigger than the battery-operated ones. The most famous and popular model used to be the Hitachi Magic Wand, which quite frankly looked like a hand blender. When I'm out speaking, I'll often hold it up and pretend to use it as a microphone. That generally gets a laugh, but hey, don't underestimate the idea of using it in role-playing. Many of the strongest plug-in models were sold in drugstores and were marketed as back massagers. Now you can find them on the internet. If you are more comfortable purchasing something that is labeled a back massager rather than a vibrator, that's fine. A rose is a rose is a rose. Or in this case, a vibrator is a vibrator is a vibrator.

One thing that may be obvious, but I'll just mention it anyhow, is that the problem with plug-in models is that they have cords and it's irritating to have a cord to contend with while you and your partner are writhing in bed. In the past few years, there has been a seismic change in this area and some extremely strong chargeable ones have been developed. There is even a chargeable Magic Wand that is extremely strong as well. So, your options are many, but for the most part, if you are having a problem, I'd start with a strong plug-in or chargeable model.

SOUND

The last thing you might want to keep in mind is noise level. Some women are really sensitive to any noise and others, less so. If you are one of those women who will start to giggle at the first buzz, you might want to consider a quieter one (although frankly, we've found that with regular use, the giggles go away pretty fast). I often have women asking me about how they can possibly use a vibrator if "my kids are in the next room." Even the big, heavy-duty plug-in ones, which tend to be the loudest, are generally too quiet to be heard through a wall or a door. I know it may sound loud to you, but try this: turn the vibrator on in your bedroom, cover it with a blanket, and go outside of your bedroom with the door closed. Hear anything? I've never had anyone tell me that they had. Next, try it without the blanket on top. This should relax you and let you use a vibrator without worrying about what your kids are going to hear.

There is also a "new-ish" type of vibrator on the market that works as a suction rather than an external vibration. They are egg shaped and have a suction that fits over the clitoris. In our experience, women who enjoy oral sex or softer and gentler stimulation seem to respond best to those vibrators. The vibrations are not as intense or powerful as their counterparts, but some women find the stimulations more satisfying and effective at helping them orgasm.

Internal Vibrators

Internal vibrators are long and thin (or at least thin-ish) and are meant to go into your vagina. Some of them are penis shaped, whereas others are not. These are vibrators you would investigate if you are interested in inserting something vaginally besides your partner's penis. This might be because you don't have a regular partner, your regular partner doesn't have a penis, or you and your partner think it would be fun and exciting to watch you put something else into your vagina. (Of course, I need to remind you that you never have to follow the rules with vibrators, and you can use that penis-shaped vibrator anywhere you darn please.) They come in a variety of shapes, sizes, and levels of realism. Here are a few things to consider:

WIDTH/DIAMETER

Some women love having something very wide that makes them feel full and even stretched. Some women don't like that feeling at all and prefer something slender. Just to be clear, even though there are some urban myths out there about wanting a "big" penis, in our experience most women are happiest and most comfortable with a medium-size girth and many find a " big" (read "wide") penis as uncomfortable and sometimes painful. So, be realistic and don't try to go after what you think you should want.

LENGTH

For the most part, a 6- to 7-inch vibrator is long enough for most women. Although the longer ones may look like fun, most women can't insert them much farther than 5 or 6 inches, so you may want to take that into consideration as well. Some internal vibrators are bendable, which can make for more comfortable insertion and use.

WATERPROOF?

If you think you'll like playing with a vibrator in the bath or shower, check out waterproof options (a significant number of vibrators are specifically made to be submerged). Please make sure you never, ever take a vibrator into the shower or bath unless it is specifically marketed to do so. You could get electrocuted, and no orgasm is worth that!

PENISLIKE OR NOT?

You'll have to decide how realistic you want your vibrator to be. Long, thin vibrators can be sleek and smooth, looking like a space-age, oversize lipstick dispenser. Or they can be shaped to look like a penis. The ones that are penis shaped can look more or less realistic, with some in skin tone shades with testicles and others in pink or purple plastic. It's all a matter of personal preference. Sometimes I'll show a patient a dildo (something that doesn't vibrate) or a vibrator that looks very realistic. She'll go all pale and say, "Ughh. Do you have something less . . . less . . . I mean, less scary?" Sometimes I'll show the same vibrator to a patient and she'll smile and say, "Great." There's no right or wrong here. It's all about how you feel.

VIBRATORS + A LITTLE EXTRA

There are also internal vibrators that are fashioned with an additional component to use on the clitoris. The famous "rabbit," as presented on *Sex and the City*, popularized these. These types of vibrators have come a long way from the first models which had clunky cords and noisy operating systems, but be wary, because they have so many moving parts (the penis and the clitoral stimulator operate separately with different speed and strength options) that they often break easily.

MATERIAL

Finally take into consideration the material of the vibrator and how it should be cleaned. Hard plastic vibrators can just be washed with soap and water; others need to be cleaned with special cleaners. Usually the websites where you purchased the vibrator will be clear about this and also have cleaning solutions for sale.

EXPENSE

In the last five to ten years, I have noticed that higher-end vibrator lines have been developed and people spend fortunes on beautiful vibrators with extra bells and whistles. If having a $200 or $500 vibrator sounds like fun to you and you can afford it, go for it. But know that if you are looking for function over form, there are probably many in the under $60 range that will perform as well for you—some of our favorites at the center are in the $20 to $30 range.

TALKING TO YOUR PARTNER ABOUT USING A VIBRATOR

My dissertation was on vibrator use by women.[1] It was a great subject for a dissertation, and it continues to be a great subject for a cocktail party. What I really wanted to look at were some of the ways in which regular women, just like you and me, reacted when they added vibrators into their sex life. What worked? What didn't work? What were our concerns? Some of the topics that I've touched on, strength, noise, and what the vibrator looks like, came from my discussions with women. But what was particularly interesting to me was the fact that so many women worried about what their partner's reaction would be.

I found that while most women said they were totally fine with talking to their partners about using a vibrator, and most of them said that they thought their partner would be really okay with the idea, most of them didn't bring it up during the duration of my study! I wanted to understand why and help them out. And, as I unpacked this issue with women, it was fascinating to see how reluctant they were. Women appeared confused, concerned, and torn about how to discuss the vibrator with their partner and how their partner might react. Here are a few quotes:

"I guess I should [tell him] because I do not usually keep things from him, but I felt like I—I guess the other thing is that I kind of did not know how to bring it up. You know what I am saying?"

"Here is my question. How do you work a vibrator into a conversation? He is sitting there and [I say,] 'I was doing the laundry today. Hey, I got a vibrator?'"

I often tell my patients, and now I'm telling you, feel free to go ahead and blame me. I tell them that they can just say that at our last appointment, we said that they should try it. And you can tell them you are reading a book that suggested using a vibrator with them, or better yet, show them this chapter. See what happens. Or just buy a vibrator, wrap it up, and give it to them as a present to use on you. Or just bring it up like anything else you would talk about. The more normally you see it, the less of an issue it will be.

On another note, women worried that their partners might feel diminished by their use of a vibrator and I think sometimes they were just transferring some of their own discomfort or questions onto their partner. Here's some things women said:

"I think he would be happier that I had the orgasm, but I think he would try to figure out what the vibrator is doing [to produce orgasm] that he wasn't."

Or "No. There are things that he is very sensitive about. I think if we had used it periodically [it would be okay], but not like every single time that we had sex. I think he would think that the thing is taking my place or she does not need me."

But here's the reality. Now having worked with hundreds of women and having spent time coaching them through both the conversation and the reality, this quote sums it up best:

"I really don't [believe he would mind]. I think anything that would give me pleasure would be fine with him. He would just be happy if I liked having sex more. Really. Also, I think it would make it more fun for him. Less work. I think it has been a little hard for him because it's gotten harder for me to have an orgasm."

Here's what I have actually found in my work with women. Lesbian and queer women seem to incorporate vibrators seamlessly. And most men (of course, there are always exceptions) are really quite okay with the idea of bringing a vibrator into the bedroom. It may take them a while to wrap their head around the idea, they may have many questions, but in the end, the honest truth is that they are usually okay with it. It's fun and a turn-on to watch your partner get aroused and have an orgasm. It's also way easier for them. Sometimes, they also feel pressure about having to use their hand or their mouth for so long. As long as it's clear that the woman is enjoying herself with them, it's all good.

Women will also sometimes say (echoing what I think they believe their partner might say) if they had the courage, "Hey, if I have a vibrator, why do I need him/her?" I'm always a bit amused by this question. Sex is not all about the physical response nor the orgasm. It's a general experience. Hopefully, an experience that makes you feel warmer, closer, and happier with your partner. I often tell women to think about it this way: Your partner could masturbate. It would no doubt be an easier and faster way to orgasm. And, honestly, sometimes the orgasms are probably more intense that way. But they want to have sex with you because sex with a partner is so much more than the mere physical components. So, yes, you may orgasm easier by yourself with the vibrator. But that is still significantly different than lying in the bed, having your partner use the vibrator on you, or using it on yourself. Your partner can be kissing you, touching you in all kinds of exquisite places, they can be fingering you, or stroking you, or talking to you. It's a different experience than using the vibrator alone. Realize and embrace that.

One of the things you do want to think about and be sensitive to, if you are buying an internal vibrator, is how your partner will react. Some partners love the idea of another realistic penis penetrating their partner's vagina. Others find it discomfiting and don't like it at all. So, you might want to discuss this issue with your partner and take their opinion into consideration if you are planning on using it with them.

Here's another question I hear: "How do I tell my partner that I actually haven't been having orgasms all this time? I mean, they think I have." It's a good question. And I know it's tricky, but I do believe, in the long run, it is a better thing to come clean about. It's hard to correct something when your partner thinks things are perfectly fine. You have a number of choices. You can come clean entirely. You can say that you love them, you love having sex with them, and you have been embarrassed to admit that you were not actually reaching orgasm. If you do that, it may sting them initially, but most adults can handle being told a truth by a partner in a loving, caring way. And though it may cause some tension, in the long run it may be very healing. Another approach that some of my patients have chosen to use is just minimizing the reality. They have approached the issue by telling their partner that they think they might not have been having full orgasms, or orgasms that are as strong as they would like, and now they realize that they are able to have strong sustainable orgasms easier with a vibrator and that they would like to try that with their partner.

However you decide to talk to your partner, you owe it to yourself to have the conversation. It may add 60 points to your sex life.

Here's an interesting story about a patient who was caught in that particular problem. When Bettina came in, she was fifty-three and had been married to the same man for thirty years. She had never had an orgasm. She was an "easy" patient, because with a little bit of coaching and the addition of a vibrator, she had orgasms easily. She was thrilled . . . except . . . except, for thirty years, she had led her husband to believe that she had been having orgasms with him. She told us there was "no way" she was going to let him know that all these years she hadn't been having one. We spent a great deal of time unpacking this and thinking about it together. She was convinced that if he knew the truth, he'd want her to have more pleasure and would be okay with the vibrator. She was also convinced that if she had more pleasure, she's want to have sex more. But she just felt stuck because she could not possibly conceive of letting him know that he'd been "mistaken" all those years.

On our fourth visit, she came in laughing. "I told him," she said. "I just out and told him. I told him I loved him and that our sex life was very important to me. I told him that I really and truly had loved our sex life. I wasn't faking that . . . just like we talked about." "And?" I said. She looked sheepish. "And he stopped talking to me for almost three days. He was furious that I had lied to him. He walked around the house moping for three days. And then, he came in and said, 'Okay. Let's see.'" She said she was stunned. "'Let's see what?'" "'Let's see the darn vibrator.'" She said she shyly brought it out and together they used it and that was it. By the time they were done, and she had an orgasm, all the bad feelings were over. "It was great! And the truth is, we're having a great time now . . . easy peasy."

So, while I don't want to minimize the issues involved in introducing a vibrator into your love life for the first time, I do want to encourage you to seriously consider it and understand that many of the obstacles that seem insurmountable may be easier to overcome than you believe. Do yourself a favor, buy a vibrator online, and boost your point profile with the click of a mouse.

CHAPTER 15

LIMERENCE, OR "SIGH. MY PARTNER DOESN'T TURN ME ON ANYMORE."

> +40 points
>
> Addressing:
>
> Primary: Desire, Arousal

There are two categories of women I see who are unhappy and feel stuck because they have little to no sexual interest in their partner: (1) women who have a dramatic "desire crash" a year or two after getting into a long-term monogamous relationship, and (2) women whose desire seems to slowly ebb and fade until they feel that it is hard to even get a glimpse of it anymore. Let's look at what a new relationship looks like, why it feels chock-full of surfeit points, what often happens over time to lose those points, and most important, how you can try to get back some of those points. Because, contrary to popular belief, you can.

You're in a new relationship. You're in love. You think about your lover all the time. Everything you do with them is special. They are your new world. Sexually, you are blissful. Even if it's not the best sex you've ever had, it's special because it's with this special person. You think about sex when you're not together. You almost never say "No, I'm not in the mood," because you usually are.

If you're someone who has always had a good sex drive, none of this feels surprising. But if you're someone who has felt that your sex drive has always been on the lower side, this may have you puzzled. It's not like you to be wanting sex this much. And you might be thinking, "I knew I had it in me. I just had to find the right person." If you've lived through this before, you may have a more depressing thought: "Early in a relationship, I want sex all the time. But after we've been together a while, I don't. It's just a matter of time. And what happens then?"

I see women in my practice on a weekly basis who are frustrated and puzzled because, early in their relationship, they wanted sex, desired it, enjoyed it, and even initiated it. Now, years—or sometimes even just months—later, they find themselves with no desire at all. They feel like there's been some invasion of the body snatchers; that some other being lived in the relationship for the first eight months and then disappeared. "He thinks I tricked him" or "I'm afraid that they think I misrepresented myself," is a common complaint. Some of the women also start to second-guess themselves, struggling to understand what it was that kept them interested in sex for those early months. They are frightened that their partner feels duped.

Most of these women's partners don't actually feel like the women set a trap to catch them, and if pressed, they wouldn't suggest that their partner pretended to like sex. But their partner is often confused and hurt by this new woman who has emerged more recently, because nothing they do seems to turn her on, and nothing they do seems sexually "right" to her. Where is the woman who couldn't wait to take her clothes off, or take their clothes off? Who moaned and sighed and was always in the mood? Partners wonder whether they have done something wrong. They wonder whether there is something they can do to change the situation. They wonder whether this is the way life will always be now.

To explain, women often create scripts to fit their new reality. "I think maybe I'm only into the chase" or "Subconsciously I was just interested in the sex because I thought I could 'get him' that way." The most despondent think, "I guess I did really trick them . . . but I didn't mean to." Women know that they felt very differently early on in the relationship, and the only way to make sense of the change is to try to provide a reason. After all, it doesn't seem normal to be a woman who wants sex one month and then doesn't a month later.

But this doesn't bear out under scrutiny. As most women describe those first months or even years of their relationship, they describe wanting sex—really wanting sex—both emotionally and physically. They don't say things like "I thought I should want sex" or "I knew they wanted sex, so I pretended to be into it." Instead, they talk about fantasizing about their lover, easily agreeing to try new sexual activities, and missing sex when they weren't having it. Many even recall masturbating for the first time in their life or masturbating more often than usual during that period. For these women, the first few months of a new sexual relationship are the most fulfilling and erotically charged; there is no hint of something calculated or altruistic involved. On the contrary, they describe it as a time in their life when they really want sex!

Now, let's look at the second group of women, those whose desire levels fall slowly, almost imperceptibly over time until it disappears. Those women's experience is less dramatic, but also devastating. These women feel that time has taken away the interest and desire that they used to feel for their partner. Boredom can set in over the years. You just finished making love and it was . . . fine. You did all the things you always like: a little kissing, a little touching, a little oral sex. You came. Then, you had intercourse, and he came. You were both exhausted, and you snuggled for a moment. But before you drifted off to sleep, you couldn't help but think, "Is that all there is?"

This scenario is also painful. No one wonders if they duped or tricked anyone, no one feels like there is something terribly wrong with them and to a certain extent people feel like this is natural: the excitement of sex falls off as time goes by. The sighs and expressions I get in these scenarios are less wrenching. But they're still heartbreaking. Because no one wants to feel like their sex life is essentially gone, over. And I truly don't think it is.

SO, WHAT IS GOING ON?

Psychologists, physicians, biologists, sex therapists, and the like can't pretend we have the whole picture of that early romantic, highly charged sexual period in the life of many a relationship. But there has been a great deal of conjecture and theorizing, and much has been written about those early stages. In 1979, the psychologist Dorothy Tennov went so far as to coin a term for the feelings and emotions that are experienced during that period: *limerence*.[1] Different from a long-term, loving relationship, this early stage is characterized by an almost irrational attachment and idealization of the object of love, obsessive thinking about the person, and a level of dependency and longing. Once the newness and all the social, physiological, and chemical rushes that come with it wear off, we've lost an awful lot of points that we had just months ago. Trying to pretend this is not the case is not only useless but can also be damaging and painful, because it forces people to try to create explanations for their behavior. "Maybe I'm out of love." "Maybe I was never really attracted to them."

Almost twenty years later, in her book *The Alchemy of Love and Lust*, Theresa Crenshaw frames this passion in a much more physical way:

Sexual whiplash is what it is. The early impulses can be so gentle you don't even notice them, or relentlessly intense, like a tidal wave. The word we call on to describe this particular magic is 'chemistry'—a perfect choice to describe a feeling that combines the giddy rush of forbidden encounter, the euphoria of an endorphin attack and the sexual surge of a street drug. All of this occurs of course without doing anything illegal, costing any money or subjecting you to any drugs—other than those you produce naturally, of course.[2]

Dr. Crenshaw sees the chemistry of limerence as the result of some combination of hormone surges (phenylethylamine [PEA], DHEA-S) and pheromones. These, she argued, are key to understanding the first flush of love and lust that overtakes us in a new relationship. Some of the chemicals are produced in larger quantities when we first meet and fall in love, some of them have the power to attract and make us fall in love, and some of them do a combination of both—a magical blend that feeds on and encourages itself. What a heady cycle we find ourselves in during those first few months!

In 2004, Helen Fisher, a noted biological anthropologist, wrote, "As you know, I have come to believe that romantic love is a universal human feeling, produced by specific chemicals and networks in the brain. But exactly which ones?"[3] Dr. Fisher's research focused more on the brain neurotransmitters dopamine and norepinephrine, as well as serotonin, a related brain chemical. The results of her brain scans of people in love are astounding. They show dramatic activity in parts of the brain that provide focus, stamina, and energy. (Remember when you could stay up all night and have sex three times and still get to work the next day? Not that you probably got that much done. You were probably still thinking about your lover.) The scans also show dramatic activity in the caudate nucleus—the brain's "reward system"—that motivates someone to general arousal and pleasure. Other researchers have suggested that early relationships also include a rush of testosterone or dopamine.

Whatever the magical cocktail—we don't fully understand it, and who knows whether we ever will—it clearly causes substantial changes in our brain, our chemical makeup, our hormone system, and our heart. The sooner we accept that there is a unique blend of emotional and chemical work going on during the early stages of a relationship, the sooner we will be able to address the problems that arise when that period of limerence is over, and we can stop blaming ourselves and our partner. It's not all bad. When the first heady rush dissipates, we can return to a normal life—less exciting, surely, but where we can get work done again.

Once upon a time, sex therapists talked about the fact that it was misleading to suggest that the eroticism left the relationship after the first few months. They were convinced, and tried to convince us, that the passion was gone merely because we didn't put enough emphasis on the relationship, and that we weren't being intimate enough with each other. We weren't communicating enough. The theory was that if we could put more intimacy into the relationship, we could also put more sizzle and sex into the relationship.

Unfortunately, this was never substantiated. It is true that if two people in a relationship are not comfortable with each other at all, or are angry at each other, they may not want to have sex or even be sexually interested in each other. But the converse is true as well. There are countless couples that go through years of talk therapy and don't get anywhere. And there are also couples who are in relationships that they would rate as good—or even better than good—where one partner just doesn't feel any sexual energy anymore.

Once upon a time, we also believed that women were naturally more suited for monogamy than men. That myth has also been debunked. Women, strikingly, more than their male counterparts, seem to have a more precipitous drop in desire for their partner as the relationship progresses![4] So, if nothing else, that should make you feel a bit better. You are not crazy and it doesn't mean your relationship is a sinking ship.

Recently a new awareness has been given to the "nonsexiness" of the intimate, ongoing relationship. In *Mating in Captivity*, Esther Perel talks about the bill of goods we have been sold regarding intimacy. "It's hard to generate excitement, anticipation and lust with the same person you look to for comfort and stability . . ."[5]

We have been encouraged to believe that the more intimate a relationship is, the better the sex will be. But that doesn't seem to hold true for many people. In reality, most couples say that the best time of their sex life was when it was new, a bit scary, and dangerous. And this is likely the key to the early sexual lust that most couples feel. The feelings at the early stage of a relationship are tied to the fear of the unknown, the excitement of the newly discovered, and the awe of the newly explored. In other words, the desire is dependent on emotions that seem to be the polar opposite of intimacy, security, and stability, and more closely associated with the erotic and the uninhibited.

"I ONLY WANT SEX IN THE BEGINNING": ELIZABETH'S STORY

Elizabeth came to see us after having been married for a year. She was thirty-two, with short dark hair, the body of an athlete (which she was), and large, worried eyes. She sat there totally still and silent for a few minutes before she began to sob as she told me her story. "I met Evan three years ago and almost from the moment we met we were inseparable. I loved being with him and we just found that we had so much in common.

"We would have sex almost every day and I was really into it, but even then, I knew it wouldn't last. The only times I seem to want sex is when I'm in the beginning of a relationship. I warned him. After we'd been together for about a year, my sex drive just seemed to gradually disappear. I told him that this is just the way that I am. I told him we didn't have to get married if he thought he couldn't deal with this. I told him I would understand. He told me he loved me, that he wanted to spend the rest of his life with me, that I was more important to him then sex."

The sobbing started again. "I think he thought it would all get better once we were married. I know he believed he loves me so much he could live without much sex . . . " Elizabeth's voice trailed off. And now, she said, he was having a very hard time. Her story ended in the way so many of them do: "I just don't know if our marriage will survive this."

Ironically, Elizabeth was still having sex with her husband twice a week, much less than he wanted, but pretty much all she could "bear." Her husband was "getting sex" twice a week, but it was pretty clear to him that Elizabeth wasn't into it, would be perfectly happy to forgo the sex, and was mostly trying to "get it over with." As much as Elizabeth was trying to be the good partner and go through the motions, she couldn't really fake it. She didn't particularly want to have sex and wasn't invested in finding it satisfying. She was doing it "for him."

MIXING SOME LIMERENCE INTO YOUR GOOD OL' RELATIONSHIP

The good news, as I explained to Elizabeth, is the fact that she reacts so well sexually in a new relationship. This would suggest that her "point" quotient is currently not so far below the threshold that she can't even access it with the rush of extra points a new relationship provides. If she was walking around with zero points, then the 40 or so points she gains from a new, hot, erotic relationship (or the dopamine, serotonin, norepinephrine, testosterone, DHEA, PEA) would not do her much good. There is something there already, all the time. It may feel dormant because she is perpetually below the 100-point threshold, but she's not so low down that she can't access it at the right moments.

This doesn't particularly make Elizabeth feel better, because one of the characteristics of hitting the "below-100 abyss" is that often, you can't imagine ever being interested in sex again. It always seems to feel as though the person who might have wanted sex at an earlier time in life was just plain someone else.

Our job was to partner with Elizabeth to figure out how to replace these points—either by working on the relationship, or through other routes.

The bad news (so to speak) is that it is very difficult to duplicate the physiologic, hormonal, and psychological rush you get from the new, edgy, and frightening feelings that occur early in the relationship. These are genuine feelings and are not easy to replicate. There are books available to help you try (and you'll find a list of them in the

Further Reading, pages 273–278). But, keep in mind, this is a hard place to garner points.

I know I said I wasn't going to give you the same advice you find in women's magazines: to role-play, to go on vacation, to watch porn. But here's the thing: when it comes to getting your sex life back on track, women's magazines aren't completely off-base. Some of their tweaks and easy-to-implement changes *can* help. Although I've already explained that something like lingerie and a hot tub can never override a point detractor as massive as pain, or that all the porn in the world won't help if your hormones are out of whack, there's no reason to leave valuable points on the table while you're resolving your issues.

But one area where magazines definitely go wrong is that they make your sex life one-size-fits-all. For some people, lingerie is just itchy. For others, candles scream "danger." Personally, I know if someone covered my bed with rose petals, all I would think about is how annoying it would be to clean up.

NOW MIGHT BE AN AUSPICIOUS TIME FOR ME TO SAY SOMETHING UNPOPULAR

Even if you have an immediate negative reaction, please hear me out and try to think about this more slowly than you might otherwise: To make your sex life work, truly work, you may have to give up some of your romantic fantasies about sex. This is difficult because, while growing up, we are given so many unreasonable visions of sex, either explicitly or implicitly, and they are so pervasive that we often don't even realize what is happening. But the truth is, we have a picture of sex that is largely spontaneous, that it "just happens." We think that we should want sex with someone we love or someone we are attracted to almost magically. We should be drawn to it, fantasize about it, and wait for it to happen "just because."

"Just because he is there," "just because we haven't had sex in a while," "just because I love her," "just because—if we are meant for each other, doesn't that just happen naturally?" And to make matters worse, those magical, unreasonable ideas got cemented early on in your relationship. During those first heady months when your hormones are raging, and your erotic sensors are heightened, and all you see is the most amazing, perfect, sexy person in front of you, it did actually work that way. You spontaneously wanted to be with that person, spend hours gazing into their eyes, cuddling in bed, trying out all kinds of sex with them, and thinking about them when they weren't around. So, yeah, "That's how it's supposed to be, right, Bat Sheva?" Unfortunately, that's not right. And while everyone is looking for the pixie dust that might make your partner crazy desirable again, I don't ever think it will exist.

What can be developed is a more grown-up understanding about sex and the role it will play in your life, in your relationship, and in your love. Now, that doesn't mean that I don't believe that magic moments can still happen in long-term relationships. They can. But they will probably not be entirely spontaneous. If you approach your sex life the right way, the grown-up way, you will be able to build and maintain a steady state of good sex. And then, occasionally, when you least expect it, you will experience those magic moments. The time when sex happened unplanned and unexpectedly or when the sex itself was just one of those explosive moments, or when you find yourself looking into your partner's eyes after sex and just feeling so warm and in love. But those moments can't happen if you are not having regular sex.

I know it's tempting to think that if you just hold off from a sex life, maybe one of those magic moments will blast through to you, but I have bad news: That just doesn't happen in my experience. It's the people with a regular, rather pedestrian, ongoing, "good enough" sex life, that turn around one day and say, "Wow. That was great sex." Or "It's great. We are going through a great patch right now."

So, what does that mean practically for you?

First of all, let's take a good hard look at your expectations. Are they reasonable and realistic? I'm going to separate between what I'll call neutral/negative and actively negative, because I believe there is a real difference in those situations. So, once again, I'm going to ask you to dive in a bit deeper and analyze your feelings. Take a look at these and think about which ones apply to you:

- I never spontaneously want to have sex.
- I never just look at my partner and want to jump them.
- I'd rather take a hot bath.
- I'd rather take a nap.
- I feel guilty that they don't turn me on.
- I love this person; I'm just not finding them sexy.
- My partner is not really my physical type.

Let's separate those from

- My partner really turns me off.
- I don't want to have sex with my partner, even theoretically. I don't particularly like them, and I don't want to be close to them.
- I really and truly would rather have sex with anyone, before I would have sex with them.

If you are in the second category, I think you may need to take a longer look at your relationship, and I would argue that this is not a sexual issue and not within the confines of this book to address. Also, if you really and truly DO NOT want to have sex, that is, you love this person, want to build a life with them, but having sex with them seems worse than going to a dentist, then you are in a different category as well. You are aversive. It's not that sex is blah, not interesting, and not magical. It's not that you are not feeling attracted to this person; rather, the idea of sex with this person makes you a bit nauseated, anxious, or panicky. If that's the case, this chapter's also not for you. You need to take a good hard look at the medication and hormone chapters (Chapters 10 and 11). The 40-point benefit of this chapter may not be enough on its own, at least not without other considerations, and the physiological elements will be critical.

But let's assume you are in the first category. You're in a relationship you want to maintain, you (usually) love this person, and you are just aggravated and sad that you don't ever seem to want to have sex with your partner. Is that you?

A MORE REALISTIC APPROACH TO A LONG-TERM SEX LIFE

First, you need to decide that you actually would like to have sex with this person. This may be a rational, in-your-head, nonmagical decision, and that may feel wrong and not like what sex is about. But it's not wrong and it's exactly what long-term grown-up sex is about. It is all about building the springboard for a good solid sex life that will, every once in a while, catapult you to a terrific sexual experience or time period.

Here's the thing: sex is a good thing.

It's good for you physically. It's good for you emotionally and it's good for your relationship. So, just as you might try to set aside time to talk to your partner, you must set aside a set time for sex. Period. End of story. And if you have sex, sometimes it will be a bit boring, but still feel good. Sometimes it will be fast and efficient, but it should still feel good. Sometimes it may make you and your partner laugh. And that will still feel good. And it will keep your blood flowing in your vagina and vulva and it will keep you connected. And it will, I hope, make you happier and it will, I hope, make your partner happier. And you know what's even better? It will set the stage for those once in a while . . . you guessed it . . . fireworks.

Once you've decided, "Okay, Bat Sheva, I get it. I should still be having sex in my relationship even if it's not spontaneous and even if it's a little draggy. I get it. Now what do I do?"

First, Schedule Sex. Period.

You need to put sex on the schedule. I don't know how to say that in a less pedantic way. But if you don't make time for sex, it just ain't gonna happen. Almost every couple I know who maintains an ongoing sex life with their partner has sex on a schedule, whether they are aware of it or not. When asked they will say, "Oh, I don't know. I guess we pretty much always have sex on the weekend." Or "Hmm . . . I don't really know, but I guess more than three or four days usually don't go by without us having sex." That's what I mean by a schedule. But if you are getting started, you might want or need to be more concrete with your partner:

"Okay, John, it's time to get our sex life back on track. Let's talk about a time that works for both us. I'm tired at night. How about Wednesdays when you work from home? Or Thursdays when you go in late? Or Saturday afternoon when the kid naps?"

I know . . . I know . . . this doesn't sound "sexy." But you need to let go of that fantasy. Just for a while. Trust me, it's way sexier to have sex once a week, sometimes by rote and sometimes really hot, than to never have any sex at all. And the starting bid for that is to set it up as a schedule.

And then . . . you need to figure out what "artificial" things might bolster you to have a regular ongoing sex life.

I'm going to give you a list of strategies. But they are all predicated on the idea that it's okay (actually it's *good*) to come up with artificial ways that make you want to have sex with this person you have chosen to be with right now. You shouldn't feel less than, you shouldn't feel guilty. You should feel reasonable, and grown up and, dare I say it, downright self-righteous that you are coming up with all kinds of ways to keep your sex life alive and breathing. Because if your sex life is alive and breathing, then sometimes it will be dancing from the rooftops. So, let's find some ways to make this work.

Fantasies—What's Happening in Your Head

The easiest approach is to use fantasies (in your head) while you are having sex or before you are having sex. Yes, you are going to have sex with the same person you have had sex with five hundred times before. But in your head, you can be having sex with three new people who look extraordinarily exciting. Or you can be ravished by the captain of the city's baseball team or you can be picked up by the sexy gal on your favorite Netflix show. You don't think you actually need to be thinking about your partner the whole time, every time, do you? Think again. There is no way any human can keep an ongoing sex life alive in a monogamous relationship without escaping into a fantasy world. Okay, maybe I shouldn't say there is no way. But I will say that it is downright unlikely.

"But that feels somehow wrong," I hear you muttering. "Isn't that kind of like cheating? And I don't want my partner thinking about anyone but me when we're having sex." At the risk of sounding redundant, I will say it again. It is time to give up on the romantic, magical, idealized, and completely unrealistic view you have about sex. "Actually, it's quite right," I'll respond. And that might be a great place to start. If you think of yourself as someone who doesn't fantasize, think again. You can learn to fantasize. It's all about learning to use your brain in a new way. It may feel awkward or uncomfortable initially, but it's absolutely critically important for you to learn to fantasize. You would be amazed at the number of points your brain can provide. Chapter 16 goes in depth as to the importance of learning to fantasize and explains to you how to do it. Get started now. Today.

The Benefits of an Affair . . . Without the Affair

When Sue found out her husband was having an affair, she was devastated. But when she comes into my office, she's also confused.

Since she found out, her libido, which had seemed to be on a permanent hiatus, has shot through the roof. They've had amazing sex four times in the last week. And it was really good sex. She is mystified and, if she is honest, she is also a bit horrified. Why should she be so interested in sex with a man with whom she is furious? She alternates between hating him and crying about him. Her trust is shot to hell. But her libido is high, and suddenly, she wants him. What the heck is going on? I'll explain this more in Chapter 17, which explores complicated emotions and how we might respond sexually in a way that feels counterintuitive to us.

But for the meantime, don't worry. I'm not suggesting you have an affair. Nor am I suggesting that you encourage your partner to have an affair. I am suggesting that we parse out elements of what happens here, and then try to use them to your advantage. Let's look at what goes through your head when your partner has an affair.

You two had slipped into a rut. You had one picture of each other and one picture only. Now, you see that guy you haven't been able to work up a lather for is maybe more attractive than you have been giving him credit for. You had been thinking he couldn't even pick up his socks, but now you realize he's capable of picking up much more than that, a new partner. And you now know there is someone else who finds him appealing and sexy.

And your competitive instinct kicks in. Wait: Why would your partner want anyone but you? You are beautiful, hot, attractive. At least you think you are, or were. What does he see in her? Well, you can do that too. What about all the things you love about him? Why are they suddenly coming into stark relief? Wait, you can keep him. You know you can.

Also, you thought you knew everything about him. But now you see you've been relying on old data. Someone else wants your partner, and you are no longer locked into your neat roles. It's a chance to break out. And even if it's terrifying, it's new—almost like you are having sex with a completely new person.

Remember how exciting that was?

Having your own affair can also juice things up in the bedroom. When you have an affair, you have a new person to fantasize about, and that person likes new and different things and introduces you to new and different things, suggests things you didn't consider, encourages you to explore parts of yourself that until now you haven't explored.

But affairs are a breach of trust. They risk your primary relationship, they are unethical, they are incredibly time consuming and often expensive. They can be dangerous if you are having unprotected sex. Also, those first heady days of high sex drive will often crash or career into serious depression or anger, and the damage is oftentimes irreparable.

So, what if you could get some of those benefits: a new person to fantasize about, getting introduced to new and different things, a person who suggests things you didn't consider and encourages you to explore parts of yourself that until now you haven't explored without the affair?

How about your current relationship?

I know what you are thinking now: isn't the advantage of a long-term sex partner the fact that you don't have to plan, strategize, worry, or orchestrate? Well, yes. But then you get to choose. You can go along without planning, strategizing, worrying, and orchestrating, but it's likely your sex life might get boring and stale. OR you can do all those things and have a fun, exciting sex life again. So, you get to pick. Isn't that great? You can ponder that while I tell you what most couples with a happy sex life do. They split their time. Sometimes they just live with the status quo and that feels fine to them at that moment, and sometimes they plan.

Mara loves her husband to pieces. He is kind. He is supportive. He is gentle. He is everything she always wanted in a life partner. But she doesn't want him sexually, at least not that way. And admitting that is one of the most terrifying things she has done in her life.

We talk about her wonderful husband, who by all she says truly sounds like an amazing person. But she admits that old boyfriends, the ones who had tattoos, who were unreliable, who took her on joy rides on their motorcycles, felt sexier to her than this lovely, kind, compassionate person. She never would have married them or trusted them or considered starting a family with them. But she wanted them.

Mara and her husband had already tried role-playing. But Mara just giggled when he tried to be the plumber who ravaged her. It all seemed so ridiculous.

I suggested we set role-playing aside and talk about finding the part of him that was harder, stronger, more aggressive in real life.

She stops for a moment and her eyes widen. Slowly, haltingly she tells me of watching him when he is working on their house, taking a sledgehammer to an existing wall, or rewiring some of their outlets. She gets turned on as she watches him work, but she feels ridiculous. It's impossible to approach him when he's working—he's concentrating hard and completely unaware she exists, which, to be honest, might be part of what turns her on. Also, she is pretty convinced that he will be irritated if she interrupts him.

I ask her to think about them when they were just starting out. If she found it incredibly sexy watching him do manual labor, would she have hesitated a minute? And if she had come on to him while he was working, he would probably have been pleased as punch, put down his tools, and gotten with the program.

So . . . here's where your attitude has to change. Your partner out of context, out of the role in which you "usually know them," is exactly what you should be looking for. These are precisely the moments to focus on elements of their personality, interests, and activities that turn you on. Don't let it be a fleeting thought. Dwell. Focus. That is how you have an affair with your partner. And if you feel shy, awkward, or uncomfortable approaching them, that's great. That feeling of taking a little bit of a risk means you are totally on the right track.

Of course, Mara and her husband shouldn't consign themselves to a life of sex only when he's doing household construction. But now they know something valuable. When her husband expresses different parts of himself, different skills or different attitudes, she appreciates it. She finds it new, and novel. It's not as simple as having your partner put on a plumber's outfit or pretending to be the contractor. It's accessing his real self—all the parts of it.

Bring-Your-Partner-to-Work Day

Role playing has its limits because, well, after all, it's role-playing. But if you want to actually access a different element of your partner's personality, you need to experience them in a different role in their life. And when women say they feel frustrated that their partner is not competent enough or they want to see a "stronger" side of their partner, I will often suggest going to their partner's office, be that a union shop, a law firm, a medical office, or a restaurant.

And I will often have women and men say to me that when they have tried this, they access a totally new side of their partner. They see someone competent, confident, liked, engaged, dressed differently, and often more put-together rather than the naggy, schleppy, sleepy person that they might normally be encountering. And that, in and of itself, makes you feel like you are with a different person.

I think it can work just as well for couples who feel that they are in a sexual rut. Move out of your normal roles and routine. You can take this as far (or not) as you like. You can visit your partner, who happens to be an electrician on a job, or the CEO of a company, and lock the door and have sex in the office. Or you can merely meet for lunch at a lovely restaurant, watch them interact with the other staff while you wait for them, and then think about them for the rest of the afternoon. Why and how we get turned on by elements of our partner's personality is complicated, mysterious, and sometimes perplexing. But it's important to keep an open mind. Chapter 17, on complicated emotions, dives into this approach and it may help you pick up some sorely missed points. Take the time to read it!

Role-Playing Lite

Sometimes people think that role-playing means full-on dressing up, meeting in a hotel, and putting on a southern accent. And, well, yes, it can mean that. And if you don't have to worry about leaving your kids with a babysitter, or that your teenager will walk in on you, then go for it.

But the reality is that there are children in the next room and deadlines tomorrow at work and you may not be up for a mock-chance-meeting at a bar in Paris. So, scale down the expectations for role-playing. Maybe use a long red wig. Or a leather jacket. Or baby doll pajamas.

Or maybe props aren't your thing. Maybe it's a storyline that you want to share. "We're both at a keg party and you see me across the room." Or "I'm Han Solo, and you're Princess Leia." Or "You're fast asleep, and I climb in the window to wake you up." Just having a starting storyline can get you and your partner thinking about sex in different ways.

Role-playing can also be as simple as remembering yourself at different times. That doesn't necessarily mean getting dressed up and going to a costume party or kissing on the subway. But what about going to a party—and secretly pretending you've just met? What about going to a bar, and having your partner try to pick you up again, like it's the first time? Simply reenacting certain parts of your relationship can bring back old feelings.

Bring Your Vacation Home

Let's face it: in that Iberian villa on the coast at sunset, the sex was hot. When you came home, it was not. But why?

People always think that what makes sex on vacations good are the classic vacation-y things: eating out every night, dual massages, sharing a shower, oiling yourselves up in the sun. And if that's true for you, too bad—you have to stay on vacation forever. (I'm just joking. Sex would get stale in the villa too.)

Some of those things do really help because they allow you to slow down, breathe, and stay in the moment. It's true that most people have better sex on vacation. But it's worth spending some time on what made *you* able to have better sex. For each person, the ingredients are different: not having a laundry list of things you have to do in your head, feeling spoiled, taken care of, pampered, feeling adventurous or just yanked out of the ordinary.

Guess what—you can do all those in real life.

Replicate the parts you like once you're home. Find a part of your city that you don't know that you can explore together. Maybe clear out a few hours at home with childcare so that you can plan out a long walk, a long bath together, and a movie in the middle of the day.

Or maybe what made you feel so pampered was not having to cook. Try upscale takeout and a movie night. Or maybe it was simply the walk in the morning that gave you time to talk, or the time alone that made you glad to see each other. Maybe it was simply an hour completely to yourselves, without internet, the kids, or the boss intruding.

Did you like a little time apart? Maybe once a month, you each get a night out by yourselves, or you make a pact that you don't have to drag your partner to the museum, or you can beg out of his reunion. Enjoyed the oasis? Set rules: no internet or TV after nine (or before nine). Liked learning something new together? Do that at home: go skydiving, buy an RV, run for office. Stasis is deadly, for your sex life and spirit.

Experiment!

A lot of the reason we're afraid of trying new things during sex is that we're afraid of looking ridiculous, and we're afraid it won't work. Well, let me break the suspense for you: when you and your partner experiment, you probably will feel ridiculous—and it might not work! You might burst into peals of laughter when your partner tries a southern accent, he might doze off at your Jane Austen fantasy. You will make each other mad and find out things that make you uncomfortable, even jealous (she's been thinking about Salma Hayek this whole time)?

As I've said, one of the things that keeps you from a healthy, happy sex life is thinking it should work perfectly all the time. But the important thing to remember is that you're together on this journey, and it's you in the room, not Salma Hayek. Trying new things is awkward and uncomfortable, but, like every other risk, it has a payoff. Believe me.

Here are some ways to break the tension:

Laugh it off. The best way to dissipate any awkwardness or discomfort is with a good old guffaw. Role-playing can be frustrating because it's play-acting. So, women in this situation will say, I just wanted to giggle when he threw me on the bed or told me he was going to "take me." That makes sense. Role-playing is fun if you both get that it's just pretending or play-acting. Okay, he looked like a four-year-old in a fireman's hat. Sure, your lingerie reminded her of her mother's nightgown. It's not personal. Share a chuckle and move on. It's tempting to be insulted that he isn't into your Princess Leia costume. Go into this open to the amusement and laughter that might ensue.

Have an open mind but feel free to nix things. This is easier said than done. But there's a reason people keep fantasies private: they can be cloaked in embarrassment, worry, even shame. Fantasies are weird: that's why they're fantasies. Use your experiments to dissipate those feelings, not aggravate them. There's a fine line between trying something new and feeling forced to try something new. But the point of this is to have fun together—not fulfill your partner's every desire. It doesn't matter if it's the fantasy they've had since high school—if something makes you uncomfortable, or seems like it crosses a boundary or hurts, say no.

Set time aside and stick to it. It's a lot of pressure to feel like you have to make life wild every other Tuesday. You also want to avoid feeling like you have to dredge up something creative when you're exhausted. Maybe set one Saturday a month to try new things, or one day a week. Or agree to just surprise each other. Either way, part of the point of this is that you're doing it together, and you want it to be fun, not a chore.

Don't Underestimate the Talking

I often hear of couples who seem mismatched when it comes to talking during sex. One of them really enjoys verbal interchanges when they are going at it. Others seem to prefer total silence. And then there is the mismatch in terms of how people want to talk. Some people want to use slang, street talk. They like the sound of "dirty" words. Others find that disturbing and like romantic interchanges when they are having sex.

It can feel pretty unbridgeable when one partner wants to scream "Fuck me harder," and the other wants to hear "You are the only one I'll ever love" in the throes of passion. Like everything else having to do with sex, preferences are individual, and it's okay to like what you like without having to understand it or explain it and certainly not justify it. But, like everything else having to do with a relationship, negotiating a solution that works for both of you is key.

In my experience, talking is one of the surest ways to relieve sexual boredom. It might involve changing the way you talk to each other. It might be by reading erotica to each other. It might be by having one person tell another person a story before or during sex.

If you're someone who likes some talking during sex, you are in the majority. Most people don't want absolute silence. If you are in a relationship with someone who seems to prefer silences here are some things to consider:

- Does your partner have no idea you want them to talk? Maybe they'd be happy to if they knew what you wanted!
- Maybe your partner is afraid of sounding stupid. Simple as it seems, the first time you let loose in the throes of passion,

you can feel very vulnerable: "What the hell did I just say???? I sounded like a porn star on steroids."

If that's the case, then you need to have a conversation where you tell your partner that (1) you are perfectly happy to be having sex with someone who sounds like a porn-star on steroids, and (2) you know it can take a while to get your verbal rhythm going.

- Maybe your partner doesn't have a clue what to say. In that case, make suggestions, ask questions while you're having sex, tell a sexy story that involves input from your partner, or read some erotica together, so they get the idea of what you're looking for.

- Ascertain whether there is some level of performance anxiety. Is your partner afraid that if they are not concentrating with all the force of concentration available to Luke Skywalker that they won't get there? If that is the case, this should be talked about and addressed in a different way. And be sensitive. Your partner might not realize this is going on.

- Take turns. As silly as it may sound, you can have silent sex night and noisy sex night. Just make sure you discuss this in advance so that everyone's expectations are met.

- If, after all this, your partner really doesn't want to talk, put an erotic show on in the background so you still have the sounds of sex, which make you feel sexy, or at the very least, consider some sexy music to use until you can work this out more.

Whether you want to talk "dirty" or romantic during sex is a matter of personal preference. I feel strongly that developing a dual vocabulary is not only good, but necessary.

Women are often scared to use "vulgar" language because on some level they have been told it's not "ladylike," or "okay." They think they will sound "dirty." But many women will express the fact that this language does turn them on precisely because there is something "bad" or illicit about it.

Many men are not programmed to talk romantically during sex. It may feel disingenuous to say, "I love you," when you're feeling "You're so hot." Some men have been programmed that talking romantically is "wussy" or not manly. But the truth is that many women will express a need for sincerity and romantic talk when they are having sex and will say that it is a big turn on. But you need to say what you want!

Caveat Emptor

Something important to think about, however, is whether boredom is truly the primary or only issue. And this goes back to something I wrote about, in Chapter 7, on low desire. Wanting to have sex with your partner should not be such hard work that you must fly to Cancún to make it happen. It's easy to blame boredom when your libido is low, because it's obvious that couples will face some level of boredom after years of monogamy. But a truly low libido really won't be fixed simply by switching things up. This can't and should not form the basis for your own points.

Think about the point system. If you are walking around with depleted hormones, or losing points because of medication or other lifestyle issues, you are going to need a LOT of points in the excitement arena to overcome that lack of points. So, if really and truly the only way you seem to want sex is with a complete stranger (add a lot of points for the unknown and the exciting) or by disappearing on a fabulous vacation (add a lot of points for excitement or relaxation or drama) or by elaborate role-playing schemes or you never, ever want to have sex again with anyone, you may want to ask yourself whether there is something more fundamental going on.

I truly believe that if you are honest with yourself, you will know whether you need 30 to 40 points that you can get by using some of these techniques or whether you really and truly are hanging really low in the point threshold and need to do something more radical, such as consider medication or hormones. And it is critical that you

remember that as you buy that red wig for you or the policeman uni-
form for your partner. Because the worst thing to do is to set yourself
up for failure.

So, consider the techniques here for getting back some of that
early lost limerence, but take a good honest look at whether or not
these extra points will really be enough.

CHAPTER 16

NEUROPLASTICITY

Change Your Brain, Change Your Sex Life

> +60 points
>
> Addressing:
>
> Primary: Arousal, Orgasm, Desire

For years, I have told women to work on developing fantasies, to read or watch erotica. I knew that it helped those women who tried it, but, like most people, I thought it just brought sex to the forefront of their thinking for the short term. My understanding of neuroplasticity has significantly changed the way that I see these exercises now. And although little research has been done on the effect of thinking about sex, it seems likely that neuroplasticity should have the same effect on sexual feelings and thoughts as anything else that comes from your brain. I have seen women adding significant points to their sex life by learning how to get their brain back in the game.

Neuroplasticity simply means that your brain can change. Maybe that doesn't sound like such a big deal to you, but until fifty years ago, most scientists believed that the brain functioned like a fixed machine. In the 1960s, a few researchers began to rethink this idea as they started to realize that individuals who had experienced severe strokes were able to regain functioning. In the past ten years, we've come to understand that the brain is much more malleable than previously believed. Recently, researchers found evidence that the brain can rewire itself following damage.[1]

We've started to understand how "plastic" the brain is, in other words, how it can grow and develop. This has had a dramic effect on how we think about changing our thoughts and behaviors. And I believe that learning the skill of thinking about sex, essentially learning to turn your brain's thoughts to sex when you want to, is key to amassing points for arousal, desire, and orgasm.

Newborns have a rapidly growing brain. At birth, we have almost all the neurons (brain cells) we will ever have, and our synapses (the connections between brain cells) are forming at a faster rate than during the rest of our life span. This makes sense because babies have so much information to assimilate in such a short period of time (What is that hand floating around and how can I make it move?). By age two or so, our brain has up to twice as many synapses as we will have in adulthood.[2] But, in a case of "use it or lose it," we lose many of those synapses as we get older. That process, in the neuroscience world, is called "pruning." By around ten years of age, we have lost about half of the synapses we had at age two because we haven't used them.[3] That is not a bad thing, because it helps our brain function more efficiently. I like the expression of "use it or lose it," because I think it pertains to so many parts of your body, your brain, your muscles, and even your vagina. If you don't pay attention and use that part of your body, it will likely either atrophy or become less functional. The more you repeat certain activities or actions, the more the brain connections associated with those actions are reinforced and strengthened. By developing new connections and pruning away weak ones, the brain is able to adapt to the changing environment.

Your brain isn't a motor; rather, think of it as a plant. How you feed and water a plant has a huge impact on its growth and development. When it's taken care of, a plant will grow larger and healthier, with more leaves. You can even direct that growth: if you want more leaves on one side, you turn that side toward the sunlight and prune away the other side. Now, think of the brain synapses as the leaves on a plant. When you want a certain brain function to work, you want more "leaves" in that area. This affects how well the synapses can communicate and form connections with one another. Everything we learn, know, and remember is due to our level of synapses in that part of the brain. Neuroplasticity suggests that you can actually develop parts of your brain, not just use more of it. You can strengthen certain parts, foster the development of more neurotransmitters (parts of the brain that communicate with other parts), change the parts of the brain that process specific types of data, and—here's where it's important for your sex life—become more responsive to certain stimuli. If you, for example, spend time doing algebra, you will no doubt expect to get better at doing these types of math problems. However, neuroplasticity suggests that the parts of your brain that you have used to work on those math problems also has become stronger, more developed, with more blood flow and neurotransmitters, and that as a result you will also become better at doing math in general, not just algebra—and you will have an easier time learning new problems that require similar skills.

What does all this mean when here you are, feeling like you are not interested in anything sexual? It means that that you can retrain your brain to get turned on more quickly, efficiently, and deliberately. When the erotic part of your brain is working smoothly and skillfully, you can call on it to get turned on when you want to—and it won't feel like so much damn work.

Understanding neuroplasticity makes me push harder on my patients who say, "I just have no interest. It's hard for me to fantasize, and I don't ever think about sex. I think I was just born that way" or "I just seem to have lost my interest sometime in the last few years." Now, I tell them, "You need to exercise your erotic brain just as you exercise other parts of your body. You need to work—hard—on that part of your brain that has become dormant. And just as exercise gets easier the more often you do it, so does learning to fantasize. I know it may feel counterintuitive. We have been told so often that sexual fantasies and thoughts will just naturally flow, they should appear out of nowhere. 'Working' on them feels absurd. But it's not. Those parts of your brain are there, waiting in the wings for you to activate them."

Because hormones affect our brain, evidence suggests a boost of them can make this process easier. This has been shown, for example, in the case of steroid hormones. In one study, when a person had a large surge of testosterone after a win, it seemed to improve their performance in later contests, which resulted in a higher probability of winning again. This would imply that hormones don't only regulate and control certain behavior, but last for extended periods and then change our future behavior and eventually our outcomes.[4] In Chapter 10, I talked a lot about how helpful testosterone can be in increasing interest and response to sexual stimulation. And there is no question in my mind, having seen it in action, that it also helps women who want to get back to using the erotic part of their brain. But the truth is, I don't believe that the hormones alone work well enough. Not without a conscious attempt to re-activate the part of the brain that manages your sexual thoughts.

There has been some current research exploring whether sex itself actually helps in the development and growth of neurotransmitters. A 2010 study found rats who engaged in "chronic" sex (once a day for fourteen consecutive days) grew more neurons in the hippocampus, the part of the brain we use for memory, than rats who were allowed only one-night stands. (I hope you find this as amusing as I do. Next thing we know, rats will be ghosting each other.)[5] The take-home message is that when you use the "sex" part of your brain, you actually are "growing" more cells in that part of your brain.

This ties in directly with sexual fantasies. It seems that when you are learning a difficult new skill, such as playing the piano, neuroplasticity even works through imagination. In 1995, a Harvard neuroscientist taught students to play a complicated piano exercise, then had them practice it two hours every day for five days. At the end of each practice session, he measured the part of the brain that controls small finger movement. Within five days, the amount of motor cortex devoted to the finger movements had spread, taking over surrounding areas of the brain. This was surprising enough. But at the same time, the researcher had another group just think about practicing the piece, doing it over and over in their mind, keeping their fingers still and simply imagining how their fingers would move if actually playing the piano. The results were amazing. The part of the brain that manages fine motor skills expanded in the imaginary players in the same way it had in subjects who had physically played the piano.[6]

FLEXING THOSE NEURONS

So, how do you use this concept to rewire, or increase the wiring, of the erotic part of your brain? How do you "practice" using your erotic brain, and how do you use the sexy part of your brain that has become "rusty" from disuse? You start focusing on fantasizing. And you do it regularly. Anxiety, the crazy pace of life, overflowing schedules: they just don't make you primed to feel sexual and probably leave you feeling that you don't really have time for this. I get it: You have the kids and their soccer practice, and that deadline at work, and the gym, and the party you are attending (or planning), and the clothes at the dry cleaner, and the watch repair guy, and the gift for your colleague and . . . the truth is, none of it can get cut. Learning to use the erotic part of your brain is not particularly time consuming, but it does mean slowing down enough to be able to experience the moment and see whether you get turned on. That, for many women, is the most difficult part. It means grabbing two to five minutes a few times a day to quiet the brain enough to switch gears. It means learning to be intentional. You will have to talk to yourself, to remind yourself to slow down enough to breathe, stop your brain from running in ten directions, and focus on thinking about something sexy. Feeling your body and brain respond to something erotic, feeling yourself get turned on can be a very slight physical feeling that is easy to miss, and if the roar of life is crashing around you, it is very likely you will miss it. But here are the techniques I recommend to my patients.

So, take a moment here. Just stop. Take a deep breath and try some of these. They are really short. They go "in between the rest of your life." Try them each a few times. And then, see what works for you:

- Get a book of erotic short stories. Stash them on a high shelf, in your bathroom or under your mattress, and then pull them out and have a three-minute read. Once you find a page or two that turns you on, put a sticky note on the page. Make a commitment to read one of those pages every day. This works especially well in the morning, because it gets that part of your brain going and more open to thinking about sex. Then, during down times, as you go about your day, your daily commute, on the subway, bus, or in your car, or while waiting for the kids at the dentist, or as you are picking up your dry cleaning, think back to that storyline. See whether you can imagine it. See whether you can get yourself turned on. One of my patients told me the best time for her was when she was making dinner. She spent a lot of mindless time, chopping, mixing, and boiling. It was a great time to put her mind to use.

   Now your job is to expand the story in your mind to make it even "better" or more erotic. What can you do to expand that story in your mind? Did you like the story of someone being watched? Imagine being watched by more people, more interesting people, in a more interesting scenario. Was there something romantic or a bit forbidden in those pages? Embroider the fantasy with more romance or more things that feel even more forbidden. This is it. You are teaching yourself to fantasize and you are exercising the erotic part of your brain. Spend a minute or two indulging in a fantasy. Let yourself get turned on. Rinse and repeat.

- Find someone cute at work, at the coffee shop, or on your commute. Watch them, fantasize about doing something sexy with that person. Or think of a really great past sexual experience you have had with someone, anyone. Allow yourself to be turned on. I know that may be contrary to everything you thought was appropriate. It's okay. Getting turned on, without expecting to do anything about it, is critically important. It's the first step to getting in touch with your sexual self. Remember, just because you are turned on, doesn't mean you need to act on it.

Evy had an appointment with us around the time that *50 Shades of Grey* was hitting its peak of popularity. She mentioned that she had bought it and was anxious to dig into it. I asked if she had read it on the train ride down. She looked at me like I was nuts. "Of course not," she told me. What was the point? Her husband wasn't with her and she wasn't going to have sex this afternoon. I laughed. "Evy," I told her, "getting turned on is not all about priming yourself to have sex immediately. You want to train your brain to be able to get turned on easily and have your body respond to your brain. The idea here is to connect with yourself and your body and to have your brain learn to do the work for you!" Again, accessing your arousal both in your brain and your body should not be something that is put in a closet until you are ready to have sex with someone. It's going to be hard to retrieve it from an overflowing closet when it's buried deep down inside. You want your sexual response to be like your favorite sweater that you whip out and wear often. Then, when it's in the closet, it will be easier to locate it because it will be sitting right on top.

- Climb into bed with your partner totally naked. Just lie there. Breathe deeply. Talk to them. Stroke their body. Lie there quietly and don't talk. Just think and be. How do you feel? If you feel yourself getting turned on, that's a good thing. You do not have to act on it. Again, the idea is to allow your brain to quiet and then to create an erotic space for you to revel in. As a matter of fact, you may decide not to act on these feelings specifically because you want to learn to allow yourself to get turned on, without necessarily having to act on it.

- When you are done working out, take a minute when you are breathing deeply to think of whatever sexy story you read recently, or the cute person you have seen at work or the coffee shop. Take a minute or two to get turned on. Some people find it easier to connect to their arousal immediately after physical activity.[7] (Many of my patients find that this is a good time to spend a few minutes fantasizing.)

- Download a meditation app. There are a bunch out there. Try "Insight Timer." Or "10% Happier." They have meditations that are 2, 5, 6, 7 minutes. Pick one when you wake up, or one before you go to sleep. Try to still yourself, if only for a few minutes. Now, once you are quieted, think sexy thoughts. Again, this is not with the idea that you are going to have sex now. This is an attempt to get your brain to focus on something sexy and then for you to be able to turn your body on by the thoughts.

OUR FANTASY ABOUT FANTASIES

Women have the misconception that fantasizing should come easily. Here's what I hear from women who often seem confused when I first speak to them. They think fantasizing shouldn't be something they have to work at; it should just "happen." I get why you might think that. There are periods in many people's life when sexual thoughts seem to pop into their head unbidden. Ask teenage boys about how often they think about sex and the answer will probably be, "Every five minutes." Some young girls may answer the same way.

When you are going through puberty and sex hormones are coursing through your body, it probably doesn't take much work to get your brain to focus on sex. But if you stop thinking about sex, or close down sexual thoughts (society doesn't help here), those parts of the brain that are used for sexual thinking get "thinned" out. Think about our plant again. There are very few leaves on those stems. They aren't going to get much sunshine in there and getting them to grow is a bit more difficult than if they were healthy and abundant. By the time you get to your therapist, that part of the brain may be stripped bare. Our job is to help you figure out how to make the plant grow again.

Another problem women commonly face when they are trying to learn to fantasize is that they naturally judge and edit their fantasies or worry that they need to share their fantasies. This is counterproductive, often unconscious, and can make it very difficult to garner points. Let's say I was trying to get you to exercise, and you go to a Zumba class. If every time you started to move, I said, "That's not right" or "You look silly" or "Yuck, gross!" you would probably go back to watching TV. The same holds true for your practice at fantasizing. If you start to get turned on by a fantasy that you think is somehow "improper" and you stop yourself, even unintentionally, you're going to impede your progress at learning how to fantasize. Eroticism is often contradictory in nature, a combination of risky and joyous, or a little scary and exciting. If you are someone who feels that you are getting turned on by the "wrong" things, take a look at Chapter 17, which talks about complicated emotions. Right now, I will tell you this: you will get the furthest in building up that part of your brain if you don't edit, don't judge, and don't get horrified by what turns you on.

Why are women so judgmental of their fantasies? The answer seems to be that lots of women are concerned that they're not "appropriate," or that they are antifeminist. "I fantasized about being overcome by a stranger in the woods." Or "I fantasized about trading sex for getting off a parking ticket from a cop." "I hate that I fantasize about those things," a patient will say. But who said fantasies should be appropriate? Not only does that sounds boring, but it's completely counterproductive. Sexual interests, or what John Money calls your "lovemap,"[9] were developed when you were very young, are instinctive, and don't necessarily make sense. They certainly don't conform to what you think of as appropriate. The minute you step into appropriate territory, you are usually walking out of the erotic zone.

People should never worry about the content of their fantasies. The whole fun of a fantasy is that it isn't real, that it isn't going to happen in real life. It doesn't reflect reality. It just means there is some element of that fantasy that appeals to you. Your job is only to identify what turns you on, not judge it! Is it the absolute power? Is it feeling incredibly beautiful? Is it a sense of equality? The romance? If you can distill the part that gets you going, you can build ever more powerful stories and images.

For instance, it is very common for women to have fantasies of being overpowered. There are any number of theories about this. Some think the appeal is that you can completely submit to pleasure when you give up control. Another theory suggests those scenarios suggest that you are so desirable, someone can't help themselves. Whatever the reasons are, being overpowered or "taken" is awfully appealing to many women. But if that happened in real life, of course you would be devastated. It wouldn't be sexy. It would be awful.

Here's something important to remember: even when you fantasize about losing control, you maintain absolute control over your fantasy. Everyone does exactly what you want, when you want it, and how you want it. You, and only you, get to decide when and how that fantasy is going to end. So, face the fact that your fantasy is just a fantasy and bears little resemblance to what you might want in real life, but if it can turn you on, you should go for it!

The most important thing for women is to enjoy their fantasies, not to feel guilty about them. What if there are two other women in your fantasy? Sixty-two people watching you? Whips and chains? A clown, an astronaut, and a person from your past? It doesn't mean that you are seriously interested in an orgy, are an exhibitionist, or are into BDSM. (Not that there's anything wrong with any of that.) It doesn't mean that you secretly want to get back with the person from your past. It just means that thinking about those things turn you on. The more you revel in your fantasies, the more your synapses will grow and, dare I say, the sexier you will feel.

Bottom line, learning or relearning to use your brain, or getting your brain back into the game, can be a powerful way to gain points. And it is a necessary part of helping yourself. Medications or hormones can help you if you are struggling with this because they can possibly make it easier to access those parts of your brain, but even when you are using those interventions, you will need to reactivate your brain and keep practicing. It is one of the most important aspects of your sexual arousal. There are no shortcuts for this and no real way around it. I know this takes work, but it is absolutely critical in the effort to regain a sexual self. So, take a deep breath, exhale, quiet your brain, start fantasizing, and start collecting those missing points.

CHAPTER 17

COMPLICATED EMOTIONS

+/− 40 points
Addressing:
Primary: Desire and Arousal
Secondary: Orgasm

Beaming, but slightly reticent, curly-haired redhead Rachel hemmed and hawed until she finally told me the problem: she wasn't enjoying sex with her husband of two years. She hasn't wanted to have sex in a long time and doesn't get turned on by him. The last part was said in a whisper, as the wide smile turned into a torrent of tears. "I can't believe I'm saying this. He's the person I love most in the whole world. He's my rock and my support." She went on to describe him to me. She said he was warm and caring, loving and sympathetic, always there for her with a cup of tea, a box of tissues, and a hug whenever she was sad. "And," she went on, "I never, ever want him to know that I just don't want him sexually anymore. I feel like such an awful person."

We talked about what gets her aroused. Although it took some time to get there, ultimately, she confessed that what she believed turned her on in the past with other partners was excitement and danger. And then we talked about what she feels most for her husband: safe and supported. I was starting to see a not-too-rare-pattern. Women talk about the fact that they love their supportive, wonderful partners, but they lust after the old high school boyfriend who rode a motorcycle and was arrested for selling drugs. But then I asked, "Does he ever get angry?"

She looked at me. Angry? And then a funny look came over her face: confusion, awareness, and a bit of horror. "Yes. Once. A year ago. He was so angry about something. And I, I was so turned on. And when he realized that, it made him even angrier." She paused and thought for a minute. "He got even angrier . . . because he works so hard to keep his temper in check. And here I was turned on by the part of him he was working so hard to erase."

Yes, there can be anger with sex. And there can be sex with anger. And there can be eroticism in danger, in narcissism, egotism, shame, power, and ruthlessness. Reaching down into the deep recesses of our emotional experiences, whatever they might be, and allowing our partners the freedom to do the same, might be one of the most helpful ways for us to reclaim our sexual desire.

Most of us believe that staring into our partner's eyes as we contemplate our love for them is the gold standard for lovemaking. Anything that falls short of "romantic" sex is subpar, even unhealthy: quickies, sex that is significantly focused on our own gratification, absent-minded sex, rough sex, sex that taps into scary emotions, sex that is "too" intense, aggressive, angry, or thoughts that we think of as shameful, seem dangerous, problematic, and dysfunctional to us. That kind of sex, we think, needs to be harnessed, rechanneled, even eradicated. But the truth is, we lose our erotic selves by trying to whitewash our sexuality or rid it of all its complicated emotions. Jack Morin, one of my all-time favorite writers on sex, suggests that difficult emotions are often some of the strongest catalysts for eroticism. His book, *The Erotic Mind*, posits the great paradox of sexuality: how shame, guilt, anger, and anxiety, often thought to be inhibitive of good sex, can turn out to be powerful aphrodisiacs.[1] Morin used data from over 350 respondents, and decoded descriptions of over one thousand peak erotic experiences. He found that many people had their most powerful sexual encounters when they were in contact with a wide assortment of emotions. He discovered that often people found sex was hotter when it was dynamic and unpredictable, rather than static and safe. Unfortunately, that is something that is difficult for many of us to acknowledge.

Morin is also the first writer I know to define the love/lust split that is so central to the work of what we, sex therapists, do. Here's the difference between love and lust: Love is an intricate and complicated tapestry of feelings: respect, concern, support, understanding, and appreciation, to name just a few. Lust, by contrast, is quite a simple emotion. It's a visceral, almost physical longing for someone sexually. And on its own, lust may work quite well in specific types of relationships: one-offs, friends with benefits, and short-term trysts. On its own, though, it usually doesn't bode well for ongoing, meaningful, long-term relationships. It's hard to sustain a relationship with a one-dimensional base and nothing but physical interest in each other to cement the relationship. But it's also difficult to sustain a long-term romantic relationship without it. You know when you hear someone talk about not being "in love" with their partner, even though they "love" them? Or when someone talks about a relationship being supportive and loving but "we feel like roommates?" What they are saying is that the lust is gone! That is a problem—and it's a more common problem than you think.

Here's the interesting thing, though: when relationships first begin, there is often an almost perfect fusion of love and lust. That is why romantic relationships oftentimes start off so heady. Oh my g-d. This person whom you love is perfect. They are the epitome of everything you have been dreaming of. And they are worthy, oh so worthy, of pursuit. And lo and behold, this perfect person is also a very sexy, desirable person. And wonder of wonders—they want you! You! What could possibly be hotter? It feels like a miracle that you found each other!

Then, the relationship continues, and something shifts. When relationships that are lustful morph into long-term, meaningful relationships, many of us start to trade in the whirlwind feelings of lust in favor of shiny romance. Why is that? Well, because deep down in our communal psyche, we really and truly believe that lust is bad, evil, and wicked. "Romantic love," on the other hand? That's noble and worthy and it's what the princesses always want in the Disney movies.

I see all around me how scared we have become of strong, carnal desire—lust with complicated emotions. We think of it as evil, wanton, uncontrollable. Sometimes it is. Hooking up or just fucking someone for fun without any thought for the needs of the other can leave a trail of destruction, not just for the other person, but also for the one initiating. Unconnected, completely thoughtless sex on a regular basis is usually not good for anyone. And for those of us in the field who have seen people pursue that type of sexual fulfillment, with no understanding of what they are doing and no checks or attempt to temper it, we know that type of sex can be concerning. We worry that when sex is only about lust and personal desire and does not consider the other person as a human being or take into account the complicated realities of human relationships, it can be dangerous. But on the other hand, we are doing terrible damage to our sexuality when we reject "lusty sex" because of a fear of where it will lead.

And we do exactly that all the time. In *Mating in Captivity*, Esther Perel makes the case that it is easy to lose the lust when we are so focused on creating intimacy and safety in a relationship. Safety and intimacy suggest that we "fuse" in our relationships and begin to think of ourselves as one unit. It's comforting to believe that we totally know our partners, totally get them, that we move in unison and there are few surprises left. That makes us feel connected. But fusion and connectivity don't create a good environment for lust to grow. The more we focus on the safe, regular, connection of love, the more we lose focus on lust, to the point where lust starts to feel, dare I say, inappropriate in our long-term relationships. Isn't that ironic?

Sex therapists could argue, and do, over the perfect combination of love and lust in any romantic relationship. Should relationships be 80/20, 50/50, or 20/80? But what any sex therapists worth their salt are clear about is that, somewhere, lust still has to exist. It's not a bad thing, it's critical to the ongoing health of the sexual relationship.

When couples come in who are totally enmeshed, totally happy and compatible, each other's best friend and snuggle bunny companion, but complain that they don't have a sex life, it doesn't surprise me at all. There is little that sex therapists agree on but I think we all agree that there needs to be some lust/love split. And most of us will agree that there is no one formula that works for everyone, but if the lust has been completely traded in for love, you have got a problem.

This fear of difficult emotions is harder for women than men. Deep down in our cultural psyche, we believe that it may be normal for men to want sex without emotions, or sex that can be angrier, objectifying, edgy, or shame based. But women? Culturally and socially, we have been taught that women really and truly cannot and do not get turned on by those emotions, that they only feel sexual in romantic, dreamy, idealized settings. And we women are the losers. Because, in my experience, many of us do get turned on by "complicated sex."

In his book *What Do Women Want?* Dan Bergner uses interviews, data, and current scientific research to help us reconsider long-held notions about female sexuality:[2]

> Women are supposed to be the standard's more natural allies, caretakers, defenders, their sexual beings more suited, biologically, to faithfulness. We hold tight to the fairytale. We hold on with the help of evolutionary psychology, a discipline whose central sexual theory comparing women and men—a theory that is thinly supported—permeates our consciousness and calms our fears.

What *do* women want? What actually ignites the lust in most women? Obviously, that is a complicated question and each woman is an individual, but I do think there are common themes that speak to many women and I think complicated emotions are often the bearers of additional points.

NARCISSISM AND OBJECTIFICATION—
BUT ONLY BY AN "ALPHA" MALE

Do we need to look any further than the overwhelming success of the *50 Shades of Grey* trilogy? I can't count the number of women who showed up in my office wanting to talk about how much these books turned them on, and how it seemed to reignite desire for those who hadn't felt it in ages.

Why is that? What turned on the hundred million readers?

There is little that is romantic about the relationship in the books. It focuses heavily on bondage and domination. But I think that might be addressing the issue too narrowly. Here's what I believe is going on. Women (and men) are turned on by being wanted. Desired. Desperately needed. We are wildly turned on by the notion that our unique, magical sexuality is irresistible. We want to be desired so much that our lover goes crazy for wanting us. And here's the rub, though: often when our regular partner pursues us, we find it irritating, annoying, like a mosquito that won't stop. So, here's what you should keep in mind. We want to be wanted and to be so hot and desired that a partner has to have us. But for many women, it's only a turn-on if it's radiating from an "alpha," someone we deem superior to us, someone "worthy," someone who can have anyone, but wants us. We don't want to be wanted by someone because we're convenient, because we're comfortable, because we're around. And it's definitely not a turn-on to be pursued by someone we find inferior to ourselves or not objectively desirable!

I don't have direct data on this. I do have the glimpses into psyches of the hundreds of women I speak to, and the picture began to converge for me when I read the absolutely brilliant book, *A Billion Wicked Thoughts*. In 2011, neuroscientists Ogi Ogas and Sai Gaddam used available data and online searches to understand not what women and men *said* they wanted and were searching for . . . but what they really wanted and were searching for. It's pretty mind-boggling because it turned on its head much of what we believed about people's sexual desire. The truth is, it's really hard to get reliable data on sex. People don't like answering questionnaires about such a personal issue, and if they do, they lie. They don't just lie to the interviewer; they lie to themselves as well. But people's searches on the internet don't lie, and by analyzing the sexual searches and by identifying who is searching for them, we can see what they are actually searching for sexually. (For example, if we know that people searching for a specific sneaker, video games, and music are seventeen-year-old boys, we can see what they are actually searching for sexually.)

When Ogas and Gaddam looked at women's searches, they were not struck by the fact that women did not consume traditional porn. That was no surprise. But the number of women who did flock to romance/sexual stories was. The number of women who read romance stories equaled the male online porn viewers! (So much for women being less interested in sex.) And what did they find in the romance/sexual stories that women did read? "One of the most fundamental and influential psychological cues for women is irresistibility: the feeling that you are sexually desirable."[3] *A Billion Wicked Thoughts* goes on to make the point that "over the past decade, sexy vampires, lusty werewolves, and a wide variety of supernatural beasties have replaced mere mortals as the most popular romance heroes and heroines"—precisely because they are "these supernatural males, alphas among alphas."[4]

Two psychologists, Maryanne Fisher and Tami Meredith, analyzed the titles of 15,019 romance novels published from 1949 to 2009 by Harlequin, the world's largest publisher of romance novels.[5] Their list of the thirteen most common hero professions in these titles included cowboys, princes, doctors, soldiers, kings, and sheriffs: "In romance titles on Amazon, there are 415 millionaires, 286 billionaires, and 263 sheiks, including *The Millionaire's Secretary*, *The Billionaire's Virgin Bride*, and *The Sheik's Secret Harem Girl*. In our own sample of 10,344 digitized romance novels from 1983 to 2008, there were no heroes who were kindergarten teachers, janitors, or accountants—except a lone accountant hero in the 1983 novel *Reckless Passion.*"[6]

Next stop: 2011's *50 Shades of Grey.* Christian Grey had cars, apartments, helicopters, fabulous wealth, and good looks, and he could have had any woman he desired, but he desired HER. What could be more of a turn-on to a woman than a man who can have whomever he wants, but he wants her!

To make my point, for it to be a turn-on, we have to be wanted by someone who, we feel, has sufficient value to be worthy of pursuit! And what the research shows is that women want to be wanted. Pretty narcissistic, if you ask me. We want to be desired, but we want to be wanted by someone who can have anyone he wants. Frankly, that feels a bit shallow, doesn't it? Bad news. Your erotic mind does not really feel particularly beholden either to political correctness or your deepest values. It just doesn't. It has a mind of its own. And what's worse is that the kind of being desired I'm describing comes pretty close to what we usually call being "objectified."

Now, let's talk about objectification. The beauty industry is growing faster than ever before. According to Business Insider, the beauty industry is valued at an estimated $532 billion internationally, and counting. Let's be honest. We're not spending that money to become more spiritual and holy. We're spending that money to look attractive, and yes, sexy. It embarrasses us to admit this, especially us feminists; but for many of us, it is a turn-on to be so attractive that we are the object of desire. Unfortunately, an additional complicating factor is that to be desired like that someone has to "externalize" us, to recognize the desired one as the other—and that takes a certain amount of objectification. But often, we hate that this turns us on. We think it's silly and shallow and . . . honestly, dangerous. And it can be. And yes, it's complicated! But it doesn't have to be. So, let's just back up a minute.

Most women do not want to be treated as *merely* a body or as an object devoid of feelings, thoughts, values, needs, and desires. It deeply bothers many of us when messages in popular culture suggest that our bodies and our sexual selves are all that matter and are valued. I'm in the front line of that revolt. However (here's where you need to think outside the box a bit), that doesn't mean that there can't be times and moments in our life when we like to be objectified. When objectification takes over our life or societal expectations, it can be a really terrible thing. But when objectification lives within a breathing, living, mutual loving relationship, it may actually function as a good thing. It's good; it's just complicated.

Here's another complicated piece of the puzzle: We are loath to acknowledge how much a turn-off it is to some women when their partner seems hurt and needy when it comes to sex. We don't want to admit to ourselves that the neediness of a partner is a turn-off, that what we experience as "pathetic neediness" for affection sometimes can make us viscerally repelled rather than aroused. But it makes a certain amount of sense, doesn't it? If a person needs us so much, then they lose a certain amount of value. It goes back to the old Groucho Marx line: I don't want to belong to any club that will have me! Suddenly our spouse feels more like a loser than Christian Grey. That's not good.

And then, in addition to being turned off, we hate ourselves for the coldness and disdain that we feel. We can feel cruel and superficial and judgmental and often confused by our "old-fashioned" ideas about sexuality.

This might be one of the hardest things for patients to admit to me. That they find their partner's desire for them "pathetic" and "needy" when he's so damn nice. All I know is that I see it again and again, this terrible cycle of the excluded partner who feels confused, rejected, lost, and terribly lonely and the partner who loves them but finds herself uniquely turned off by the neediness.

I also know that it's terribly hard to work your way out of that place. Sometimes I just want to tell a husband: "You know what? Tell her 'screw you.' There are a bunch of women out there who find me attractive and wonderful. You are an idiot for not seeing it. I'm done. Call me when you are ready to actually work on the situation." Ironically, that might alleviate the problem. But these partners, like you, are stuck in their current dynamic. These husbands are also caught in a situation where they have been told that unconditional love and support, patience, and expressing sad emotions are the gold standard they are supposed to live by. What these partners may not always understand is that "expressing their emotions" also needs to include the stronger emotions, such as impatience, aggression, and anger. But that's obviously much more complicated and scarier. If you feel like this speaks to you, you might want to have your partner read this part of the book.

COMPETITIVENESS

Early on in my practice, I had a wonderful, smart, gutsy patient trying to recover from her husband's affair. She was typical of a woman dealing with the aftermath of her spouse's infidelity. She had bouts of hope and bouts of depression. She struggled to rebuild trust in her relationship. But she also took it as a sign to attend to her sex life, which had be faltering for many years. She wondered often whether the affair was an outgrowth of a sexual problem, or whether it had caused it. But she noticed that, counterintuitively, her husband's affair had actually increased her sex drive.

This scenario repeats itself again and again with numerous patients; it's not such an isolated or unusual reaction. Your partner had an affair. It's out in the open, and you know about it and are furious, hurt, and wounded, or even when you don't know, you just suspect something is going on. Some women respond in a way that might seem more intuitive to us: they are furious and hurt, and they can't imagine ever having sex with their partner again. But many women respond to the news of their partner's affair in a completely opposite way: they find that it ignites their desire and they want to have sex more than they may have for years. We'll often have women saying to us, "I hate myself" or "I am so totally confused, but since I found out about the affair, suddenly my libido is back!"

I think there are two things at play here. One: these women's newfound sexuality is partially due to their finding out, deep down, that their husband is truly independent and separate individual from them. They understand, in a fundamental way, that much as they truly would like to believe they know and understand everything about their spouse, that is not true. And, honestly, they may never know him entirely.

That's painful. But it also adds a small layer of mystery and possibility to the relationship; it's also sexy, because we don't really want to have sex with someone who is so familiar to us. We want to have sex with someone new and exciting and different. That's why the sex is often best early on in a relationship. And why it feels like a challenge to keep the spark alive when you've been with someone for a long time. Old cozy socks are not sexy. The new shoes in the window . . . more so.

Here's the second reason: an affair also means that someone else finds this man sexy. We are a herd species; we often value what others value, even if we think it's silly to do so. That's how crazy styles take hold. If everyone else thinks ripped jeans are attractive . . . well, you guess they must be. And they start to look so much better than they would if you just saw them in isolation. So, if someone else thinks your partner is sexy, sexy enough to have a sexual relationship, you find yourself taking a second look. And maybe for the first time in a very, very long time, you look at this man and see him for how he is seen by someone else. And you know what? He looks pretty good.

So, when an affair catapults you into seeing your partner as a separate being, and someone who is attractive to someone else, it really is no longer crazy or surprising that it might ignite your desire. As I watch my patients struggle, I want to reassure them that they are not crazy; rather, this might be information that they can use in the future.

SHAME

I have a patient who gets turned on by shame. And the shame she feels by getting turned on by shame puts that shame to shame. She doesn't want to get turned on by shame, by fantasies of being talked down to and scolded and told she is no good. She had a complicated and borderline-abusive relationship with her extended family as a child and she often wonders whether that is where it comes from. Maybe it does, but that doesn't change the reality that now her most powerful fantasies are of shame.

The world of sadomasochism (the SM in BDSM) is pretty popular. Around 11 percent of the population are willing to admit that they actively participated in S&M, and 5 to 7 percent say that they regularly include verbal humiliation into their sexual activity, women more than men.[7] Honestly, I believe that statistic is a low-ball number, both because who wants to admit to an interviewer that they want to be shamed in a relationship, and because my patients' experiences tell me otherwise.

I know that there are therapists who feel that my patient would need to work through her history to scrub clean the shame. I don't know. In my experience that might take years, and I am skeptical as to how successful she'll be. And I'm not sure why we need to be judgmental of people's erotic catalysts. Women sometimes like to be called a "bitch," a "slut," or a "bitchy slut," and we should stop shaming women who like to be shamed. It's their right. But that doesn't seem to work well in our current cultural narrative that seems to think that because sex has to be consensual it also has to be vanilla. My favorite quote from the BDSM community is that BDSM must be based on consent. Otherwise, it would be . . . abuse!

In this scenario, my patient's choices are limited. She can try to cut off the shame-based turn-on. That's hard to do. After a time, we are pretty hard-wired. Or she could own the shame as an adult, possibly resetting it somewhat, and use it as a tool to enjoy her erotic experience. Maybe that means having a partner who says shameful things to her before they make love or asks her to crawl across the floor to get his clothing. You may want to think of this as a type of role-playing, and it can be. But it can also be a mutually consensual time when she is allowed to own the emotions that, while turning her on, are not healthy or effective in the rest of her life. If both she and her partner are turned on by her shame-based fantasies, then I say go for it. And after they have great, hot, erotic sex, they shift off their sex personalities, and he reverts back to the respectful partner who takes in the dry-cleaning, does the dishes after dinner, or brings her coffee in the morning. And really, what has been lost?

ANGER 2.0

But what about Rachel and her husband? And his fear of showing anger and her fear of responding so strongly to it? This is a classic dilemma: A couple gets married and then each begins molding the other to better fit the relationship and the perfect human they want to be with. They start to slowly "shave away" some of the uncomfortable, complicated emotions, even though they might be the exact same things that turned them on initially.

I see it all the time. I see it with my own relationship, with my friends' relationships, with my clients' relationships. We pick someone often precisely because they have specific qualities that viscerally attract us. They are independent thinkers. They don't really care about other peoples' opinions. They take over a whole room. They are loud and funny.

Then, we live with them. Or marry them. And suddenly, some of those strong independent qualities don't look so good anymore. They are hard to live with. And so we go about, subtly, or not so subtly, scrubbing them clean of exactly those qualities that turned us on initially, whether we were aware of it or not!

And then, we wonder what happened in the bedroom.

Anger is the classic emotion that couples try to eradicate. I commonly see anger being "scrubbed" from relationships. Most of us think of anger as scary and dangerous. We are afraid of anger. Especially in our modern-day liberal world, we leave little room for anger.

Let's remember that anger is one of the most basic human emotions. Tied to the sympathetic nervous system, and the "reptilian brain," it allows us to consolidate our energy quickly and efficiently to respond to perceived problems. It's present in the most primitive part of our brain and the same part that connects us most primally to sex. As in other areas, the same emotion that, unconstrained, can be destructive and violent, when managed and channeled appropriately, can connect us most viscerally to our body and our experience.

Anger is just one of many of our strong emotions that make us uncomfortable, and as a result, we banish from our emotional repertoire. And I think our attempt to rid our partners of any intense emotions, but specifically anger, may be backfiring.

NOW, WHAT?

One of the things that bothers me is that the same books that have done a great job defining the problem don't do much when trying to offer solutions. But it's really hard. I need to acknowledge that adding points here is complicated. This is not quite as straightforward as "stop taking this medication" or "add this medication" or spend ten minutes a day fantasizing. This is a place where you really have to find your own way. Yes, one solution is to move on to a new partner who you haven't scrubbed clean of all the scary emotions that make you uncomfortable outside the bedroom but who turns you on in the bedroom. But that's not the solution I think you might be looking for, at least not those of you interested in a long-term monogamous relationship. Another solution couples use is to open up their relationship to additional sexual partners. Not a bad idea, either, but one that often doesn't appeal practically or ethically or otherwise isn't acceptable to most of the women who come to see me.

So, what's our solution? How do we garner points in a world that is so complex, where cultural mores are amorphous? I know it's hard, but it's important that you are honest with both yourself and your partner about what turns you on and what turns you off. First, you have to identify those things. You need to stop and take a while to figure out what it is that is turning you on. It might be weird, unexpected, and maybe even . . . may feel wrong? But, as I tell my patients, when something feels risky or scary, that is often a good sign that they are on their way to an erotic encounter. Then, here's the harder part. It might mean fessing up to your partner that:

- You love them, but you have lost connection to the lust you felt for them.
- You get turned on by things that might feel sketchy to you or to them or to both of you.
- You feel the need to free up both of you, to explore parts of yourself that might feel scary or that would be distasteful in other parts of your life.
- That shaming or being angry and ruthless would be a turn on, or their opposites—being shamed, scolded, or managed.
- That guilt can sometime turn you on.

If watching your partner play tackle football turns you on, think about who they are when they are playing and see whether the two of you can figure out a way for them to tap into that part of themselves. Imagine this conversation:

"But, honey, I feel ruthless when I play with the guys. I'm aggressive. I don't give a shit about anything but getting that ball over the line and I will mow over anyone in my way to get it."

"Yes, dear. And that is precisely what is turning me on."

"But isn't that . . . objectifying you?" Horror overtakes your partner's face.

"Maybe. And maybe sometimes I need to be objectified by you to see you deeply turned on, and for me to be truly turned on. That doesn't mean I want you to be that way all day long. I would hate that person during the ongoing routine of my life and that of my kids. But can you find that person in the bedroom?"

Some of you are thinking, "I can't possibly do that. I've been married for twenty years to the same person and we know each other so well. If they showed up tomorrow and I was wearing black leather and holding handcuffs, they would think they came into the wrong home. And I'm not sure I could stay with the strong controlling part of me that wants to tie them up and make them beg for sex."

Or you might be thinking, "Really? What is going to happen to my relationship if, the next time we have sex, I tell them to call me a slut, tie me up, and make me beg for sex; ask them to slap me or humiliate me or control me? Are they going to think I have lost my mind? Will they file for a divorce from this new crazy woman who has invaded their home?"

Here's my response: You don't actually know whether you can pull it off until you try. Even then, like any other change, it takes practice. You may be quite surprised by the result. Your partner might get turned on, really turned on. But what's significantly more important is that you might get turned on, more turned on than you have been in years. Allowing yourself to experience the complicated emotions that live deep within the recesses of your psyche might allow you to experience lusty sex again, and isn't that worth the small risk involved in your relationship?

Understand that doing something sexy and dangerous could be as benign as moving your own hand onto your own clitoris during intercourse. Or it could be something more edgy, such as seating your partner, tied up across the room in a chair, while you perform a slow striptease. When a patient says, "I couldn't possibly do that. I'd feel so awkward, so . . . slutty?" I tell them that delving into the dark side is often ever so much hotter than safely staying with the light.

As Jack Morin put it,

> Whenever you deliberately introduce an element of raunchiness into an encounter or fantasy, some of your enthusiasm comes from a subtle undercurrent of guilt, perhaps recalled from an earlier time. Chances are you won't be thinking about guilt consciously because you have succeeded in neutralizing its negative, inhibiting qualities by taking control of it, claiming it as your own, and mastering it by using it for your own sexy purposes. Your disobedience becomes a demonstration that your desires are superior to the pitiful prohibitions that dare to dampen your enthusiasm. Guilt reveals its richest aphrodisiac potential when it is not forgotten, but vanquished.[8]

There might be the part of you that slips out of a friend's party into a back room to fool around. It feels a bit foolish, right? You have a house you live in and a bed you are both in every night. That's so easy. But this is different. Entirely different. You feel a bit naughty and scared, which triggers a whole bunch of emotions: shame, daring, risk. These all bump up your erotic response. And yes, you run the risk of getting caught by your host, but so what really? You're together. You're legal. The worst they can say is that your sex life is out of control. Not the worst thing for someone to think, is it?

Rachel came back in a few sessions later. She was amused and a bit embarrassed when she described a tryst she and her husband had at her in-laws. She had literally yanked him into the bathroom for sex. She was laughing as she told me about how squished they were in the ground-floor powder room. But then, something else crossed her face as she described how, at first, he thought she was crazy and was laughing. But when he realized that she was serious, how incredibly turned on he got, and how hot the sex had been. She stopped and was quiet for a minute. We both knew that she understood what I had been getting at. The powder-room sex had been quick and fast and not particularly emotional. It was her doing what she wanted with him. And in doing so, she had freed up both of them to respond erotically. Now it was her job to figure out how to allow some of that back into her marriage on a more regular basis.

Using a specific element of our partner's personality to help us explore our erotic turn-ons doesn't have to change, or even touch, our day-to-day experiences with the person. It doesn't have to reflect the rest of our relationship—in fact, maybe it shouldn't. But it also isn't "role playing" as we commonly think of it. We aren't each pretending to be something we're not. I am describing something more real than role-playing. I'm describing getting in touch—or back in touch—with the parts of your partner that turn you on and allowing them to exhibit deeper, darker sides of themselves.

So, go. Embrace your emotions in all their wild and crazy variations, and in the process reclaim those hefty amounts of points that have gotten lost in the loving relationship. Embrace your partner's emotions and allow them to express the wide range they may have, and trust that your relationship will be better for it.

CHAPTER 18

MEN ARE FROM MARS.
MAYBE YOU NEED TO EXPLORE MARS.

> *+60 points*
>
> *Addressing:*
>
> *Primary: Desire, Arousal, Orgasm*

D elilah sat in my office across the small table. "We are not having sex anymore, and it's all my fault," she said. "I've never had particularly good desire. I've never initiated. And now we are not having any sex at all."

Her words sounded awfully familiar, yet something about what she said about being the lower-desire partner brought me up short. I've learned over the years to ask more questions in those cases, so I did.

"Was there a time where you initiated more? Was there some rupture or significant change in the relationship?" I was getting only nos. She wasn't turning her husband down, and her desire level hadn't changed all that much over the years. I stopped to think, and reframed.

"So, you are telling me that you never had much spontaneous desire, but most of the time when your husband approached you for sex, you were happy to go along with him. And for twenty-seven years, he's been initiating, and you've been responding, and your sex life has been okay. And now, somehow you are not having sex at all."

She nodded, holding back tears. "Delilah," I suggested, "could it be that all these years your husband has been the 'engine' of your sex life pulling you along, and now that he's not initiating, there is no engine for the train?"

Her eyes got wide. "But if he's stopped initiating," she said, "it's got to be because he got tired of being the engine, of the fact that he had to always initiate sex. My low sex drive has turned off his desire."

There was silence for a minute while I weighed my words: "Maybe," I finally said. "Who knows? But could it also be that his desire has dropped for some other reason that truly has nothing to do with you? And with no engine, that train is just not going anywhere?" I continued carefully: "Delilah, as a betting woman, I'd hazard a guess he just didn't wake up one day after twenty-seven years and become turned off because you didn't initiate."

She looked skeptical. "Don't get me wrong." I continued. "If your level of sexual interest isn't working in your relationship at the moment, that can and should be addressed. I just think it's possible his not initiating may have to do with something with him that you absolutely aren't responsible for, like lowered hormones, depression, stress, or a million other things." There was quiet as we both sat there. She opened her mouth a few times as if to argue, but then just started crying. (That's why I have a box of tissues on my table.)

If there is one thing I've learned in my practice over the years, it's that we women—most of us, at least—blame ourselves. For everything. What's crazier, we invent a scenario that overlooks more obvious possibilities or sidetrack potential explanations to stack things up in a way where it comes out to be our fault. And that is why so many women come in saying, "We're not having sex. And I know it's my fault."

Taking all of the responsibility may seem noble, but it's not particularly helpful because it often means we miss obvious solutions. I also think there is a less altruistic explanation for why we women are so quick to blame ourselves. If it's our fault, it is more likely we can fix the problem. If it's someone else's, we have no control. The problem might not be able to be fixed.

Take Delilah. If the problem is hers, then she can simply begin to initiate. But if the problem is her husband's, then what? She might have to convince him to get help, or deal with his resistance or denial. If none of that works? She might have to live with the problem.

It's critical that you are honest about what is going on with your partner so that the two of you can address the issue together. Otherwise, you can't solve the problem. After all, Delilah's husband might be willing to do some work to help improve his libido. Or it might take work on Delilah's part to change the part of her that was always working as the body of the train rather than the engine. Realizing what is going on does not necessarily absolve Delilah from doing her share, but it takes away the false relief of thinking everything is in her control and she can fix everything herself. And while that may be painful, it is also more realistic—and more likely to help solve the problems.

Social constructs seem to have done a number on both men and women, telling us what "all women are like" and "what all men are like." And there are cases where that can be helpful, which may be why *Men Are from Mars, Women Are from Venus* was such a popular book. But when we start with preconceived notions that may, or may not, be relevant to the men in our life (if we have men in our life), it can have significant ramifications on our sex life. Understanding the male perspective might be quite helpful in gaining you some sorely needed points.

Listen: Men have it tougher than we think. Hear me out.

Recently, I was speaking to an all-male class of rabbinical students. I said in passing that I think we do a disservice to men in our society by assuming that they are, or should be, always in the mood to have sex. It seemed to resonate strongly. Basically, it caused a small commotion. "Thank you for saying that!" one guy said. "Sometimes I'm not in the mood to have sex, and when that happens, I start to question my own masculinity. What the hell is wrong with me? Don't all guys want to have sex all the time?"

The truth is, men don't "always want to have sex," and to suggest it is just as harmful as declaring that women are never in the mood.

The students were tremendously relieved to hear someone from "the other side" see it from their point of view. It hit me that, in trying to be helpful, we unwittingly put a lot of pressure on the guys in our life.

Here are some myths about male sexuality I'd like to bust:

1. **Men always want/look for/are ready for sex.**

   I am always amazed at the number of women (generally those with a low libido) who tell me they think their husband would only truly be happy if he was having sex every day. Once we've gotten their libido back to normal, I give them a challenge. I suggest that they initiate sex every night for two weeks and see what happens. Never fails: by week two, the husbands say something like "Again? Honey, I'm kind of tired."

2. **Men are not picky. They'll have sex with anyone, anytime.**

   This one really gets me. For many men, the most important part of sex is the emotional connection. If they wanted just a physical release, they could masturbate, and forget about the mess and fuss. But they don't. They want to be with you. Many women connect by talking. But many men connect by doing. That's why you often hear of women meeting to have coffee and talk, but often men will go "do" something: fish, play basketball. In my experience, for many men, the act of having sex with you makes them feel close and connected. That's why you might want or need to talk things out to feel more loving toward him, but he might want to have sex to feel more loving toward you.

3. **Men are not interested in the other physical connectors, such as touching, kissing, cuddling.**

   Perhaps the most poignant thing I hear from men whose wives suffer from low libido is the dual sense of loss they feel in their relationship. Not only have they lost the sexual activity, but they've also lost the closeness and the touching that they need. And often they are not imagining things, or wrong. The women are afraid if they kiss, touch, or cuddle, when they are not in the mood to have a sexual rendezvous, that their partner will take that as a signal that they are in the mood and try to have sex. But the male partners talk so sadly about how much they miss the physical connection in its entirety!

MAKING CONTACT WITH MARS

I highly recommend, if you feel like something is off between you and your male partner, that you sit down and try to talk about it. More important, that you sit down and ask questions, and actually listen to what your partner is saying. Try not to make a priori assumptions about what is happening. Here's some concrete advice about how to have this conversation:

- Don't do it at a time that is linked to sex: when you just had (bad) sex, when he turned down your approach, when you are heading home from a date night, when he just distanced himself emotionally.
- Find a neutral time and place, ideally away from the bedroom, where there is ample time to talk and no distractions to allow the conversation to get waylaid. The car, a walk or hike, a trip to a store.
- Start by communicating your love (even if you are angry and hurt) or describing what the relationship means to you (even if that feels silly when you've been together for twenty years and doesn't he know that already?).
- Express what you are experiencing, not what you think or believe is going on (using "I" statements, at least when you start the conversation).
- Be willing to make yourself vulnerable by expressing your honest emotions. I'm guessing, even if you are experiencing anger, that is probably coming from being hurt, confused, lonely, or afraid. Those emotions are the real ones and those are the ones you might want to express first.

Here's an example: "Honey, I need to talk to you about something [preparing him for the conversation]. I think you know how much I love you [expressing your commitment and appreciation], but I'm feeling really hurt and confused right now [expressing what you are feeling]. Our sex life seems to have disintegrated recently. I mean, not that we were ever the sex pistols, but we used to have sex once or twice a week and it was pretty good. At least I thought so. But we haven't had sex in three months. It feels like you are often tired, or just not interested [describing your experience]. Have you noticed this also [No accusations, just an open-ended question]?"

Here's a word of caution. These conversations are often not one-time discussions. Sometimes, women find that their partner is (or feigns to be) clueless. He hasn't "noticed" that his interest level has dropped. And maybe it's true that he hasn't noticed because denial is a powerful stress management tool, or maybe he has noticed but he hasn't connected the dots for himself yet. He is having erection issues and he didn't realize that affected his desire. Or he thought maybe it was just the new job or whatever. So, often this will be the first conversation of a few.

These are hard conversation to have because, whether we are aware of it or not, wanting sex from someone who seems uninterested is an incredibly vulnerable position to be in. It is critically important, that as bad as you feel, or as hurt or abandoned or angry, that you don't get accusatory. That will just make matters worse. Whether it is fair or not, because of communal expectations, it is significantly more difficult for a man to come to terms with the fact that he is not functioning sexually. And frankly, it's not so easy for us women to accept that is true about us either.

The truth is that once a man starts to look more objectively at his sex life, the disparate pieces might start to put together the puzzle for him, and you. And most of the men in a committed relationship do want to have the relationship continue. So, have a first conversation, and maybe a second or third, and maybe even suggest that he read this chapter. It might help shed some light for him on what's going on.

COMMON PARTNER PROBLEMS
THAT TAKE AWAY POINTS

Here are the things that come up all the time in heterosexual relationships. And when they do, I really encourage you not to ignore the
issue but discuss them "early and often" and not put them off until
someone is feeling terrible and too many secondary problems have
been created.

Erection Problems

Erection issues can be a result of nervousness, stress, and performance anxiety. However, for most men over age thirty-five, there is
primarily a physical reason, which can be vascular, neurological, and/
or hormonal. Fortunately, with the right help, if a man has a penis,
he can get an erection.

But we women are quick to assume that we are a big part of the
problem.

Let's think about this scenario, and let's use the 100-point model
to put it into perspective. A fifty-eight-year-old man comes into the
office because he is having a difficult time achieving an erection with
his wife. He is beside himself, because when a thirty-five-year-old
manager, from another department, came onto him at the holiday
office party, he got an erection in thirty seconds flat. He didn't do
anything about it, but he certainly felt like he could have.

Now, he is feeling horrible about his relationship to his wife,
whom he loves, and thinks is very sexy, even after thirty-three years.
He must be not attracted to his wife anymore, right?

Wrong!

All the scenario means is that he seems to need a higher level of
erotic stimulus to get an erection. Think of our 100-point model . . .
again. (Yes, our points model applies to men as well!)

Our fifty-eight-year-old may get turned on by his wife's kisses
and touch, but he's only at 70 points before she starts. Her caresses,

though fun and stimulating, may only give him 20 points. A thirty-five-year-old he barely knows, on the other hand, is erotic and new, which provides an extra 50 points. That may blast him up to 120 points. No problem with the erections now.

But his logical, conscious brain doesn't want to have sex with a fellow employee. He wants to have good sex with this wife. So, that just means that we have to find a way to get him an additional 10 points with his wife. It may be fantasy. It may be medication. It may be a change of scene. But it doesn't means he needs to be with someone new.

When our male partner has trouble maintaining an erection, our first thought is, *I bore him. I'm not sexy enough. Is he having an affair?* But this is needlessly painful. And, in addition to sending us into a negative spiral of blaming ourselves, it is also uniquely unhelpful.

Say your partner just started high blood pressure medication. Suddenly, he finds himself having trouble maintaining an erection. Your first thought, no doubt, is not to consider what medical changes have occurred recently with your partner. Your first thought is that you're the problem. And so, rather than having a forthright conversation with your man, you decide to fix yourself. You buy over-the-top lingerie, come onto him directly. He tries to avoid sex because he's insecure about his erections. You think it's you again and try harder. He gets panicky. He starts getting angry at you when you initiate. Now, you're alarmed. He must be having an affair! And now you're panicking.

What could have been a fifteen-minute conversation turned into a full-blown crisis. Ideally, you could have sent him back to the doctor to change medications or get treatment. Or you could have just had nonintercourse sex to take the pressure off. But, by blaming yourself, you did neither of these things, and because you two aren't having any kind of sex at all, you feel awful about your sexuality, and he feels like a loser.

Life doesn't get easier when you take everything personally. So, rather than thinking of yourself as the "root" of the problem, think of yourself as providing "less points" than he needs, now that he has changed physically, or the relationship is less new. Take a step back and assume it's not you for five minutes. "Honey, I've noticed that we haven't had sex in a while, and that the last three times we tried to have intercourse, your erection wasn't so strong. Has something changed?" If there are no drug changes, or major life stressors affecting your partner, then it's probably time to get a physical evaluation. Sometime erection problems can be an early warning sign of larger medical issues, but for the most part, they are just related to age, blood flow, or hormone levels. And they can be fixed. So, don't panic. Don't blame yourself. Don't go into a crazy tailspin. Sit down and have a conversation, make a medical appointment, and fix this problem as you'd fix any other problem. If you stop seeing his erections as a commentary on your sexiness, you'll have a much easier time addressing issues in a helpful way.

Premature Ejaculation (PE)

This is the term we use to describe a man ejaculating before he (or you) is ready. And like problems with erection, it can be tied to anxiety, but not always. It can be severe enough that he does it while you're fooling around, or at first thrust. Then there are some men who can hold off their ejaculation for a few minutes, but it takes intense concentration. And it's incredibly frustrating for both of you. You can spend a lot of time blaming yourself, feeling that you must be doing something wrong, or, if you have less experience, feeling that this is the way intercourse always is.

The most useful definition of premature ejaculation I have heard comes from our center's medical director, Michael Werner. He taught me that the best way he determines whether someone has premature ejaculation is by seeing whether his attempt at holding back his ejaculation is taking up too much mental space during sex. So, if, when you have intercourse, your partner is always saying, "Wait, don't move. Okay, you can move . . . Oh, no. Wait, stop. NO,

STOP!" he probably has premature ejaculation. I can't tell you how many women I have seen who are convinced that their partner's PE is their fault. It isn't.

Some men have lifelong PE. For these men, it is almost always biological. It is simply the way they were born. It is not a psychological problem or learned response. Although it will always be the way he is built, it can always be managed. His ejaculation can always be delayed by pills, topical anesthetics, or behavioral changes. Or his erections can be managed so that he keeps it after ejaculation and can continue having intercourse.

Some men develop premature ejaculation after having good control previously. This is often related to having erection issues or other sources of anxiety. Often, when the underlying issue is addressed, a man will regain better ejaculatory control.

The great thing about PE is that it can always be managed!

On the other hand, the stress of one person feeling bad about themselves and the way that they have sex can wreak havoc with a sexual relationship. Men can start avoiding sex or blame their partner. This can have a serious ripple effect in the long term, taking away points that you need. Don't take this on yourself. Talk it out with your partner and try to find a specialist in male sexual dysfunction. Barring that, try a urologist. That is always a good starting point.

Low Desire

Your partner doesn't want sex. And you don't really know if your partner doesn't want sex or doesn't want sex with you. This can be devastating. There is something so fundamental and elemental about being wanted by your partner. And when that is gone, people of both sexes describe a horrible void, and an incredible sense of rejection.

Just because your partner has no sex drive doesn't mean that the problem is you or that they find you less desirable. I want you to repeat that to yourself ten times. I have spent hours sitting with women helping them to understand the pain their lack of desire is causing their partner. I try to help women see that for their partner sex truly goes beyond being able to "get off," and is often directly linked to feeling connected, desirable, and "wanted." And this is just the reverse. The same is true for you.

Low desire may be the most insidious of all partner problems, because it makes us feel alone and unlovable, even when the problem really is not directly related to us. And figuring out whether your partner doesn't want sex at all or just doesn't want it with you, is honestly a very difficult conversation to have. But have it you must, if you want to fix the problem.

In my experience, if the problem is a general diminishment of desire and not a direct response to your relationship, your partner will be quick to say so and often very vociferously. The exception, however, is that your partner himself is confused about his lack of general interest in sex and embarrassed about it. In that case, he might not want to talk about it. But please understand this: if your relationship is basically okay, then it's most likely that the low desire has to do with stress, exhaustion, age, medication, hormones, erection issues, or a combination of those factors, and is not directly related to you.

Of course, there is always a possibility that he may be having complicated feelings about you, or may be too involved with porn to want sex with a live woman, or may be having an affair. Unfortunately, those are questions you really can't answer without talking with him. If that feels too difficult or scary a conversation for you to have alone with him, you may want to see a couple's counselor to help you untangle the question. (For more on therapy, see page 255.)

It is, however, truly important to know that, just as a woman's libido can be helped through a combination of lifestyle changes, medication adjustments, hormonal therapy, and behavioral changes, so can a man's. Low testosterone can wreak havoc with a man's libido and is very common as men get older. And with a good medical care provider, a bit of time, patience, and support, your man's libido can be up and running before you know it. And you may even get your engine back! Which, can, of course, be a big points-booster for you.

If you are having problems that seem to relate to your partner's sexual functioning, here are some summary guidelines:

- If the problem seems to lie with your partner, and not you, it probably does.
- Don't always put the blame on yourself. It helps no one.
- Don't assume that you can fix these problems for your partner. That also helps no one.
- Sit down and ask questions as nonjudgmentally as you can. Listen well. That will help.
- **Almost every one of these problems can be fixed with help.** So, get the help you need, be it a therapist, a medical practitioner, or a combination of both.

A NOTE OF CAUTION IF YOU DECIDE TO GO THE COUPLES COUNSELOR ROUTE

If a primary reason that you are going to see a professional is because your sex life has disintegrated, you need a couples counselor who is educated and comfortable talking about sex. If you see a therapist and they say something to the effect of "Let's get your communication fixed and then the sex will fix itself," run for the hills. Unfortunately, there are couples counselors out there who are not really equipped to deal with sexual issues. Some of them are aware of that and don't take on those cases; others are not self-aware enough to make that call. And there are others who truly believe that the sexual relationship will follow the emotional one. I believe they are wrong. I think it is perfectly possible that a couple gets along well, doesn't argue, has great communication, and still has significant problems with their sex life.

It's perfectly okay if a couples therapist says that they want to get to know you for two or three sessions before jumping into your sex life, or if they say, "I think you are both angry at each other and here's why and I think we need to address that while we are dealing with your sexual problems." That's fine. Sexual problems are complicated and are most often intertwined with other issues (either because they are a result of those problems, or because they caused them). However, a good couples counselor should be able to encourage you to talk about your sex life, or lack thereof, and shouldn't allow the topic to move off center stage unless they have explained to you exactly why it has not been addressed in that period of time. If you do decide to go the counselor route, be sure to check out Appendix II, page 271.

And there you have it. Your partner's sexual problems can take away a whopping 60 points. And it can feel hopeless because you can't necessarily fix them yourself. But with the right help and guidance, you should be able to recapture those points.

CHAPTER 19

GO THE F*CK TO SLEEP

Sex with Children in the House

> + 20 points
> Addressing:
> Primary: Desire, Arousal
> Secondary: Orgasm

Mothers of newborns are exhausted. They are sleep-deprived, overtouched, and often feel as though they are dripping from every orifice. They don't feel sexy. They often don't feel that they look sexy and often they can't imagine ever feeling sexy again.

Parents of toddlers are often exhausted as well. Whether you work outside the home or spend your day with your child, running after a preschooler is like running a marathon, except there are too many interruptions to allow for endorphin production. And then there are the going-to-bed rituals, which can involve ten trips back and forth to someone's bedroom and often one parent falling asleep with their child.

Older kids bring their own challenges. Somehow, they're now more interested in your life and your bedroom. Drawers and closets that you thought may be off-limits get rifled through, and wandering visits at night can become the norm.

Then, they become teenagers. Finally, they put themselves to bed. But now you realize—gasp—they stay up later than you do. And who in the hell wants to have sex with your kids sitting outside your door? It puts a crimp in your moaning and groaning.

When my kids were teens, I got a birthday card from my husband that described the situation perfectly. The first panel had a picture of two teenagers sneaking off to the basement to have sex while their parents watched TV in the next room. The second panel had a picture of two middle-aged parents sneaking off to have sex while their teenagers watched TV in the next room. It said, "The years go by, but not much changes." Having sex when you have kids is a big challenge, and it lasts as long as they're in the house. So, what's a person to do?

Here's the deal: Staying long term in a marriage is hard. Staying on the same page as your partner when you are raising kids is hard. Staying united as a team when you are raising kids is hard. Staying together fifteen years later when the kids leave and you are back to being just two again (yes, trust me, that day will come) is perhaps the most difficult challenge of all.

But sex makes that easier. And it makes it easier because it is the glue that holds you together, the thing that marks this relationship as more than just a cooperative. If the sex in your life is good, you should be able to laugh together, hold each other through difficult times, and know that there is someone who has your back. And a good sex life with your partner will make the difficult child-rearing years so much easier for you as a couple.

POSTBIRTH, IS THERE A HAPPILY EVER?

You *know* you used to be into sex. Yes, that was you, not someone else. But it just doesn't seem to be happening that way anymore. You have this fantasy that it will all go back to normal once your kids hit the next phase, but it doesn't.

Many women find that their libido drops dramatically after the birth of a child. This may not happen after the first or even the second child. Some find it drops after number three, or four. Some have the problem after each of them. They are tired and stressed. They don't have enough time to take a shower, let alone have a sexual rendezvous with their partner.

But you want to have sex again. And you want to solve the problem. So, here's a broad list of factors that can be at play.

- **You *are* probably tired and stressed.** Taking care of children is more work both physically and emotionally than we ever anticipate.
- **You may be *"overtouched."*** Who wants to have their nipples fondled after they've just spent the morning breastfeeding?
- **Your self-definition may have changed unconsciously (or consciously).** Hey, you are the mother of three now. Is it really okay for you to also be the babe who comes into your husband's shower with two glasses of wine, or screams dirty things as you have an orgasm?
- **You children are becoming sexual beings.** How could you possibly have a child that old and what the hell do you know and what should you be telling them? Or you may be just a tad bit jealous of the kids who are just starting out their sexual life when yours seems to have hit a dead-end.
- **You may be angry at your spouse.** Perhaps you are upset that more responsibility for the house and the kids seems to always fall on you. And then they expect you to do what?? You may not be outwardly angry, but maybe angry enough that it is affecting your desire to make love with your partner.
- **Your hormones likely have shifted significantly.** Two stages here—first, during your pregnancy and postpartum; second, later in life. The labor, birth, and possibly an episiotomy may have created subtle (or not so subtle) physical changes that seem to make it harder to get aroused and have an orgasm. Or it's later in life and you are so busy shepherding kids to soccer practice that you don't realize that you've hit forty-two and are heading into perimenopause. Discomfort and pain are big obstacles on the road to romance.
- **It may not be the childbirth at all.** It may be your age, changing blood flow, or irregular hormone levels. I know our

kids keep us young, but unfortunately, they don't freeze us in time!

- **You're out of practice.** Oddly enough, sex seems to feed on itself. The more you have, the more you want. The less you have, the less you seem to think about it.
- **Maybe you need a different kind of sex.** Your life has changed significantly. Maybe those two-hour lovemaking sessions are a thing of the past (for right now) and you are having trouble adjusting to a fifteen-minute "quickie."

FOR ALL PARENTS WHOSE SEX LIFE SEEMS TO HAVE DWINDLED

The first step is to sit down and ask yourself honestly what you believe is going on. Make a list of all the factors that you think are impacting your libido. Try *not* to make a list of things that "should" or "might" be affecting your desire for sex; rather, those things that ring true for you. Are you exhausted all the time, pissed off at your husband, and feeling queasy about feeling sexy? Or do you feel like yes, you are exhausted, but you suspect that there is something physiological going on? Women often have a good idea what's really happening when they are able to have an honest conversation. Sure, you could try harder. But you can't, or you would be.

Here are some things you can do to get things back on track:

- **Sleep more.** Yes, I know. This is every mother's dream, but sleep deprivation messes with your hormone levels and, as a result, your mood, your patience, your ability to see things clearly. Before you consider hormonal intervention, see whether there is anything at all you can do to get more sleep. Maybe letting your partner know that more sleep for you might lead to more sex for you both will be a motivator. Or hire a sitter. I know it sounds crazy to pay for a nap, but it isn't.

- **Exercise**. I'm sorry. I know that, like sleep, lack of time is the biggest obstacle here and that most moms would give their right arm for a few hours of sleep and time at the gym. However, like sleep, exercise helps balance your hormones. It has to become a "must" rather than a "like." Which leads me to my linchpin argument . . .

- **Get childcare help.** I'm suggesting getting more support because the odds of your getting more sleep, exercise, or couples counseling without getting more help is ludicrous. And at the risk of sounding like Marie Antoinette, I get that more help may not sound financially feasible for many people. But if you need to, consider stopping the investments in college briefly and invest in your sex life. (Divorce is expensive!) Try to form "help exchanges" with your partner and friends (if you're tired and have no time, your friends probably are as well): You watch the kids for two hours while I go to the gym, and I'll keep the kids for two hours so you can sleep.

   I remember when I was pregnant with number three. It was five in the afternoon and I had gotten off work early. I knew if I went home, I'd end up playing with my kids or taking them out. Instead, I showed up at the door of a dear friend and asked if I could crash on her couch. She didn't make me feel silly and she didn't try to talk to me. She walked me over to the sofa, told me to knock myself out. Which I did, literally. I woke up at 6:30 p.m. feeling like a new woman.

- **Get housekeeping help**. It sounds so absurd for a sex therapist to strategize with a patient about cleaning, laundry, and folding, but I find myself doing just that during many appointments. Of every other aspect of life that can probably be addressed, this is the most basic and easily accessed. If it's at all financially possible to get help, even sporadically, in this area, go for it and don't feel guilty. If you have friends or family who can help out (yes, also even sporadically), call in those favors. Because I am telling you that it's worth the investment in your relationship. And, because it is often a bone of contention between couples, it avoids stress too. Another, less expensive option, is for you and your partner is to make a decision to learn to live with a messy house for a while.

- **Have a heart-to-heart talk with your partner** about what is going on. They are probably also stressed, over their limit, and ready to explode, but for them, it is very possible that sex is a stress reliever and now they want or need sex more. For you, it may not feel that way; rather, it is more likely another source of stress.

  Sit down. Talk about the fact that you are not having sex. See whether together you can create a concrete plan for carving out more time for you to sleep, exercise, and have sex. I am not minimizing the amount of creative thinking this takes. Nor am I discounting the fact that having that creative thinking while you are in a sleep-deprived brain fog is difficult, but if you want to fix the situation, that should be your starting point. If you feel that a therapist, life coach, or even a financial planner might be helpful in sorting all of this out, then reach out for them and get help.

BOUNDARIES IN THE BEDROOM

Ah, your bedroom. The bedroom is for cuddling, it's for watching television, it's for hanging out with the kids, it's for getting dressed and for conking out. Remember what else it's for? Sex.

Every month, another women's magazine has an article about how you should "make your bedroom an oasis." Or "keep the bedroom for sex." And when I see this, I have a difficult time stifling a snort.

For most women I know, the bedroom is the newest form of the multipurpose room. But I do think that you can and should create boundaries for the bedroom that allow you to convert it into a good place to have sex when you want to.

You'd be amazed at how a little bit of management can make your busy bedroom more conducive to sex. And while that doesn't solve a low libido problem, it can address the "I have trouble getting in the mood" problem.

Try the following:

- **A lock on your door.** Many parents have kids that wander in at night and they don't make their bedrooms "off limits." There does, however, have to be a level of security that allows you to relax when you are having sex and not have to wonder all the time whether you will look up and see a small head peering down at you asking what you and Daddy are doing.
- **A white noise machine.** This can be a fan turned on in your bathroom or an actual white noise machine, but either way, you need something that allows you to relax and not have to whisper when you are having sex, especially with teenagers in the house. White noise machines are inexpensive and easy to find.
- **A small or diffuse light source.** Most people have a bedside lamp or something that allows you to have sex without the overhead light making you feel that you are in a gym or in pitch darkness. Good lighting also affects your mood.
- **A place to put the family pet outside of the bedroom.** I am sorry. Having a whiny, jealous pet or a furry face coming between you and your lover is not a way to make sex more erotic. Believe me, they will love you anyhow.
- **An easy-access sex towel**, or something to put under you for those wet spots that invariably happen. I know, wet spots are not "talked about," but let's face it, sex can be messy. And knowing you have a sex towel in easy reach, to put under you when you have intercourse or to wipe up ejaculate, will make rolling over and cuddling easier. While you're at it, make sure you have a box of tissues handy for the after-mess as well.
- A **private closet or drawer** within easy reach to store lubricants, vibrators, sexy books, or whatever other accoutrements

you and your partner like. This might mean putting a lock on your nightstand drawer or just keeping a locked box somewhere near the bed. It takes a little bit of planning, but it really makes a big difference.

PUT SEX ON THE FAMILY CALENDAR (NOT LITERALLY, PLEASE)

This is an idea that I've stated numerous times in this book, but it bears repeating here. If you want a sex life that withstands the years together, the births, and the raising of children, you will have to give up some of those fantasies of spontaneous sex. Likely, it might not happen. Or it might happen. But if it does happen, it will be on special, rare occasions. And the best way to encourage it to happen on those special, rare occasions, is to have a regular, ongoing sex life. And that, as unromantic as it sounds, takes decisions and planning. So, the best way I know to keep your sex life alive with your permanent partner is to plan both the regular sex dates (or as one of the therapists in my office calls it—naked time) and the once-in-a-while-remember-how-great-our-sex-life-used-to-be dates. And both of those take some effort and some energy.

You and your partner should probably have a conversation about a reasonable frequency of regular sexual activity. This needs to be direct and clear (hinting or subtle suggestions get lost between diaper changes, school form signatures, and hockey practice). Try:

"Sweetie, sex seems to have gotten lost in the last year. I think we need to think about carving out 'us' time, both to connect and to have sex. Wednesday during naptime? Thursday morning when you are working from home? Saturday nights when the kids are all out? Let's just set up a specific time for us to have sex each week. I miss having a sex life with you!" Talk about it, make a decision, and try hard to stick to it.

Then, once a year (or dare I even suggest twice a year), see whether there is any way to go away with your partner. I know it's tough. But if possible, I think it's worth it. So, find a parent, a sibling, a sitter, or even friends you can trade off childcare with. And pack those bags and go. You don't have to go far; you can even go to the motel around the corner, but make some real, uninterrupted quiet time for you to reconnect. I always suggest, if possible, two nights. The first night, people just crash. No matter how sex starved they are, they are usually more sleep deprived.

When you are most disconnected, most down on the relationship, most aggravated at your partner, that might be the most important time to go. I remember one time, years ago, my husband and I were not in a great place emotionally. We were all set to go away for four days. It took a mammoth amount of planning and organizing, which of course, fell on me. I was resentful, irritated with my husband, and exhausted. I complained to my friend Sari that my husband was the very last person I wanted to go away with. "Why don't you just come instead?" I whined. She started to laugh and said, "When your husband is the LAST person you want to go away with, that is exactly when you need to go away!! So, shut up and go." And she was right, of course. I did. And I came back feeling very differently. It was a good lesson for me to learn and I've truly internalized it. Relationships are hard work, and if you and your significant other are merely working as business partners and operations managers, it becomes really, really hard to remember why you chose each other in the first place. And having quiet time to spend together is a basic prerequisite for reconnecting. So, carving out real time together, and sex as a part of that, is an important ingredient to making things work. It's hard maintaining a long-term relationship. Don't let anyone tell you otherwise.

The bottom line is that we let our kids take over our life. Even for those of us with careers we love and things we want to accomplish outside the family, our kids, by necessity, often become the center. And, as a result, our primary relationship suffers. The only way I know to guard against that, is to plan for it and to follow up.

Your relationship will be so much better off in the long run. Your point threshold will be better for it now.

CHAPTER 20

YOU GOT THIS

I t's time to put down this book and start working on your own plan. Whether that plan includes finding medical professionals to support your process, setting yourself goals in particular areas, tackling the difficult conversation that needs to happen, or buying a new toy, this is the moment to create real life changes. By now, you have figured out where you are missing points and you have had a chance to dive into those chapters that you think might be helpful in finding them. I have confidence in you and know that you can address any problems you are having.

Before I take my leave, here are some closing thoughts that I hope will make this project feel a bit less scary or daunting.

- **You are not crazy, and you are not alone.** Right at this very moment, millions of women are facing the same issues you are. I know that doesn't solve the problem, but I hope it helps you feel less isolated and out of sync.

- **The problems you are experiencing are most likely multifactorial.** That is, they most likely are not the result of one thing out of alignment. But hey, at this point, you know that already, don't you? You understand that they are probably the result of a combination of different things. Working on some of those things, even if you can't work on all of them, will make a real difference.

- **Progress probably won't be linear.** You might find that you are working on one thing, and it will go well, but then you might get stalled out for a while. That's okay. When you go back to pick it up, you won't be starting from scratch. You'll be starting from somewhere further along. And eventually that will get you where you want to go. You can also work on a few things at the same time. You're using dilators to help with the pain? This might also be a good time to start working on your fantasy life or talking to your partner about trying something outside your comfort zone. And if the dilation goes off track for a while, you can still work on the fantasies.

- **Like most other things in life, your sex life changes**, morphs, blossoms, recedes, hides, and reblooms. This will likely not be the last time you need to address sexual issues. There will be other problems along the way. That's okay. You now have the tools to fix them.
- **It may feel daunting sometimes.** These problems didn't develop overnight. And they probably won't disappear overnight. But I do promise you that if you keep focusing on the solutions, one day you realize that the problem is much more minimal than it once was. Or—and this is the real payoff—you can hardly remember that the problem ever existed!
- **Don't ever be afraid to ask for help.** Not from your health-care providers, not from your friends, and not from your partner. None of us live in isolation. Expertise, support, and encouragement go a long way in helping you to get to the finish line.
- **You can make the necessary changes.** I know you can. I have seen hundreds of women make serious changes to their sex life. I have seen them go from feeling sad and hopeless to feeling empowered and, dare I say it, happy. There is no reason you can't be one of them.

Your sexual self is worth the effort! Knowing that you own, really own, your sexuality, and can take care of your sexual self is one of the most empowering experiences a woman can have. Stand up tall. Pay attention and own your sex life. I know you've got this!

SCHEDULING SEX AND SCHEDULING NOT-SEX

There are times we recommend "scheduling" sex—and not-sex—as a way to change some of the avoidant habits that may have developed when your desire faded. It is also a great way to begin to build back in some of the physical affection that sometimes gets lost when a sexual relationship has been rocky for a while. Here are some tips:

- Decide on a schedule for specific "sex dates." In most cases, I would recommend once a week, but if it feels intolerable, start with twice a month. It needs to be a frequency that you can keep up with a positive attitude and with minimal resentment.
- Decide on **specific time(s)** (e.g., Friday nights or Saturday afternoons).
- Those times will be "sacrosanct"; they will be specific and definite.
- The "lower-desire" partner will approach the sex date in as positive and loving way as possible. *If for some reason that time won't work for logistical reasons, the lower-desire partner **has the responsibility for rescheduling another specific time in its place.***
- During the rest of the week, both partners understand *that there will be **no expectation of sex**.* **Period.** Even if the lower-desire partner engages in cuddling, kissing, snuggling, sexual talk, etc., there will be absolutely no expectation of sex by the higher-desire partner. The higher-desire partner will not assume that they are being invited to engage in sex *unless asked to do so explicitly in words* and will not try to convince or maneuver their partner into sexual activity.

THE BENEFITS

Scheduling sex (and not-sex) this way often significantly alters the sexual dynamic and has positive effects on the relationship.

- It reassures the partner who wants and needs sex, that there will be a definite time to have sex. This relieves some of the tension regarding the "ifs" and "whens" of sex. The relief in knowing that sex is coming may help a partner feel less stressed out, less irritable and lonely, and more patient and loving.
- Scheduling sex allows the lower-desire partner to return to being more loving and physical with their partner. Rolling over in bed to kiss or hug without the tension of "will my partner take this as a signal that I want sex?" is really freeing. It often allows couples to get back to physical contact and intimacy that they may not have experienced in years.
- Finally, there are times when "not having sex" becomes a habit; and changing habits, as we all know, can be very difficult. Having a scheduled time for sex helps break this "habit," and may help couples get their sex life on a new footing.

For this to work, both partners have to be absolutely vigilant about maintaining their boundaries and responsibilities:

If the person with lower desire does not approach sex in a positive, loving way at the designated time, their partner is likely to feel betrayed and abandoned, or become angry, hurt, or resentful.

On the other hand, if the higher-desire partner makes a move to have sex on a nonscheduled time, the lower-desire partner will lose trust. They will not believe that they can be physical and loving without it leading to sex and they will likely revert to their inability or unwillingness to touch and caress.

A BRIEF GUIDE TO FINDING THE RIGHT THERAPIST

Finding the right therapist can be daunting. Ask friends, family, or your primary care office whether they have recommendations. Do an internet search (PsychologyToday.com has a reference portal), read reviews carefully and thoroughly, and try to read between the lines.

I strongly encourage you to call a potential therapist and have a five- to ten-minute phone consultation before you book your first appointment. You can save yourself a lot of time and bad first appointments if you screen therapists on the phone and see whether you feel comfortable with them. If you feel you can afford it, you might seriously consider setting up two or three first appointments with several therapists. Comparison between experiences can be invaluable and in the long run might save you time and money. Here is a list of things to look for:

- **A license:** This is necessary. The term *psychotherapist* can, unfortunately, be used by anyone. Having a license does not guarantee that someone will be a good therapist, but at least you know that they've had the proper training. Look for such qualifications as licensed clinical psychologist; licensed clinical social worker; licensed clinical marriage and family therapist; or licensed mental health counselor.
- **Training in sex therapy:** Their website (or their credential when they speak to you) would include having completed any number of programs in sex therapy or they can have accreditation (not licensing) in sex therapy.
- **Specialization in one or a few specific areas:** Some therapists say that they work with couples, families, kids, stress, anxiety, body

issues, eating disorders, anger management, depression, sex therapy. It's not a good sign. Find a provider who works with individuals and couples and maybe one or two other specialties.

Here are some questions to ask:

- Where is your sex therapy training from?
  - They should be able to point to some formal training or accreditation.
- Do you have a particular approach to treating individuals'/couples' sexual issues?
  - If they say, "We work on the relationship and the sex will follow," run for the hills.
- What approaches or techniques do you use?
- How do you feel about the use of medication?
- How do you approach pelvic pain issues?

You are not looking for specific answers. Many excellent therapists use varied techniques, but a good therapist will listen to your story and address your issues without fitting you into one way of thinking or working. You also want someone who is open to any other treatments you are considering and will work collaboratively with your health-care practitioners and other therapists.

FURTHER READING

GENERAL BOOKS ABOUT SEX

Sex Matters for Women: A Complete Guide to Taking Care of
Your Sexual Self, by Sallie Folley, MSW, Sally A. Kope, MSW, and
Dennis P. Sugrue, PhD (2012)

Reflections of diverse women throughout the life span as well as
science-based information are the basis for the exercises and advice provided in the book. It covers body image, anatomy, hormones, relationships, sexual orientation, sexually transmitted infections, and trauma.

Guide to Getting It On and *Guide to Getting It On Unzipped,*
by Paul Joannides (2004, 2017)

This lively, upbeat book covers nearly every element of sexuality in a
straightforward, plain-talking, humorous way. Filled with comics-style
pictures and short sections, it is aimed at a young, hip audience, and
honestly, it's one of my all-time favorites.

Pleasure: A Woman's Guide to Getting the Sex You Want, Need,
and Deserve, by Hilda Hutcherson (2006)

A guide and intro for women in heterosexual relationships. It covers
basic anatomy, various forms of sexual pleasuring, and ideas to make
your sex life more interesting.

Come As You Are: The Surprising New Science That Will Transform
Your Sex Life, by Emily Nagoski, PhD (2015)

A fun exploration of women's sexuality, based on research and brain
science. In clear, approachable prose, Dr. Nagoski explains why there is
such a range in how women experience sexual cues and thoughts.

The Vagina Bible: The Vulva and the Vagina: Separating the Myth from the Medicine, by Jen Gunter, MD (2019)

Written by an ob-gyn with no patience for pseudoscience, this book busts myths about vulvar/vaginal health and gives you data-driven information in its mission to educate and empower.

MORE READING ON PAIN

Healing Pelvic Pain, by Amy Stein (2008)

With its focus on improving the underlying cause of your pain, this book outlines exercises, nutrition, and self-care therapy. It includes a stretching, muscle-strengthening, and massage program you can do at home.

Sex Without Pain: A Self-Treatment Guide to the Sex Life You Deserve, by Heather Jeffcoat, DPT (2014)

This concise self-treatment guide, written by a pelvic floor physical therapist, offers an approach to treating women using dilation techniques. It is straightforward and includes step-by-step guidance with clear drawings as well as exercises for large muscle groups, progressive relaxation, and treatment aides.

When Sex Seems Impossible: Stories of Vaginismus & How You Can Achieve Intimacy, by Peter T. Pacik (2010)

Written by the physician who developed the Botox treatment for vaginismus, this book explores experiences of women with vaginismus and outlines and champions the Botox injections as one excellent solution.

MORE READING ON ORGASMS

Becoming Orgasmic: A Sexual and Personal Growth Program for Women, by Julia R. Heiman, PhD, and Joseph LoPiccolo, PhD (1988)

Although some might find this book a bit dated, it is one of the classics on overcoming orgasmic difficulty. It includes an introduction to the female anatomy, relaxation exercises, and step-by-step instructions.

The Elusive Orgasm: A Woman's Guide to Why She Can't and How She Can Orgasm, by Vivienne Cass, PhD (2007)

In easy-to-read language, Dr. Cass provides a full overview of women's sexual pleasure, covering sexual triggers, stages of arousal, the power of mind, and how women differ from men.

Becoming Cliterate, by Laurie Mintz, PhD (2017)

Providing a sociological context as to why so many women struggle with orgasm, this book uses biology, sex therapy, and sociology to gives you both information and concrete advice on anatomy and how to fix the problems.

MORE READING ON RELATIONSHIPS AND SEX

The Sex-Starved Marriage: Boosting Your Marriage Libido: A Couple's Guide, by Michelle Weiner Davis (2003)

Written for couples negotiating a relationship with a low-libido partner. It outlines potential causes and suggests solutions as well as validates each partner's respective experience.

She Comes First: The Thinking Man's Guide to Pleasuring a Woman, by Ian Kerner (2008)

This book is written for partners of women; serves to help educate and guide and offer tips on pleasuring a women's anatomy.

Mating in Captivity: Reconciling the Erotic and the Domestic, by Esther Perel (2006)

A poetic read that addresses the issue of low libido. It explores why some eroticism is lost when there is a high degree of intimacy and we feel safe and secure.

The Seven Principles for Making Marriage Work: A Practical Guide from the Country's Foremost Relationship Expert, by John Gottman, PhD, and Nan Silver (2015)

The book is based on the authors' years of researching couples' interactions. The result is concrete and clear advice to help couples collaborate more effectively and resolve conflicts of any kind.

The 5 Love Languages: The Secret to Love That Lasts, by Gary Chapman (2009)

This book is small but packs a powerful punch. Chapman believes that love is a way of behaving as much as it is an emotion, and that expressing love is a language we need to learn.

Hold Me Tight: Seven Conversations for a Lifetime of Love, by Sue Johnson, EdD (2011)

This book introduces and outlines Emotionally Focused Therapy (EFT), a tool for couples working to break out of negative cycles of negative communication cycles.

MORE READING ON FANTASY AND EROTICA

The Erotic Mind: Unlocking the Inner Sources of Passion and Fulfillment, by Jack Morin (1995)

The sourcebook on erotic fantasies, both beautifully written and powerful, it explores why we have fantasies and get turned on by the things that we do.

Tell Me What You Want: The Science of Sexual Desire and How It Can Improve Your Sex Life, by Justin J. Lehmiller (2018)

Understanding how common fantasies are can ease anxiety and shame about our own fantasies. This book is based on the most comprehensive survey ever tackled on the subject.

MORE ON OVERCOMING SEXUAL ABUSE OR TRAUMA

The Courage to Heal: A Guide for the Women Survivors of Sexual Abuse, by Ellen Bass and Laura Davis (2008)

This book is a guide that offers hope and a map of the healing journey to women with childhood sexual trauma histories—and to those who care about them.

The Body Remembers: The Psychophysiology of Trauma and Trauma Treatment, by Babette Rothschild (2000)

This gracefully written book full of absorbing case studies integrates the physiological research of trauma into treatment.

The Body Keeps the Score: Brain, Mind, and Body in the Healing of Trauma, by Bessel A. van der Kolk, MD (2014)

In this triumphant book, Bessel van der Kolk explains how trauma affects brain development and attachment systems. He gives us a fusion of clinical cases, neuroscience, and humanism to heal trauma.

MORE READING ON HORMONES

Estrogen Matters, by Avrum Bluming, MD, and Carol Tavris, PhD (2018)

Far and away the best overview available on the history and use of estrogen. This book is clear, readable, scientific, and myth-shattering as it outlines the history, concerns, and benefits of HRT.

The Secret Female Hormone: How Testosterone Replacement Can Change Your Life, by Kathy C. Maupin, MD (2014)

This book shares research on the symptoms of aging that are initiated and accelerated by estrogen and testosterone loss, including mood swings, changes in sex drive, and general health.

The Female Brain, by Louann Brizendine (2007)

In a highly accessible way, this book explores both brain chemistry and hormones to better explain the unique brain-body-behavior of women.

The Menopause Book: The Complete Guide: Hormones: Hot Flashes, Health, Mood, Sleep and Sex, by Pat Wingert and Barbara Kantrowitz (2018)

Comprehensive and informative, this guidebook separates menopause fact from fiction. It is divided into sections to ease your read.

Our Bodies, Ourselves: Menopause—Boston's Women's Health Book Collective (2006)

This book both delivers important information and women's personal stories. Its mission is to help us become more comfortable with menopause and better educated when considering treatment options.

NOTES

CHAPTER 4

1. M. A. Lahaie et al., "Vaginismus: A Review of the Literature on the Classification/Diagnosis, Etiology and Treatment," *Women's Health* (London) 6 (2010): 705–719; I. P. Spector and M. P. Carey, "Incidence and Prevalence of the Sexual Dysfunctions: A Critical Review of the Empirical Literature," *Archives of Sexual Behavior* 19 (1990): 389–408.

2. Peter Pacik, "Botox Treatment for Vaginismus," *Journal of the American Society for Plastic Surgeons* 124, no. 6 (December 2009): 455e–456e, https://doi.org/10.1097/PRS.0b013e3181bf7f11.

CHAPTER 6

1. Elizabeth A. Lloyd, *The Case of the Female Orgasm: Bias in the Science of Evolution* (Cambridge: Harvard University Press, 2005).

2. R. J. Levin, "Sexual Activity, Health and Well-being—The Beneficial Roles of Coitus and Masturbation," *Sexual and Relationship Therapy* 22, no. 1 (November 2006): 135–148, https://doi.org/10.1080/14681990601149197.

3. J. E. Frank, P. Mistretta, and W. Will, "Diagnosis and Treatment of Female Sexual Dysfunction," *American Family Physician* 77, no. 5 (March 2008): 635–642.

4. C. M. Meston and B. B. Gorzalka, "The Effects of Immediate, Delayed, and Residual Sympathetic Activation on Sexual Arousal in Women," *Behavior Research and Therapy* 34, no. 2 (February 1996): 143–148, https://doi.org/10.1016/0005-7967(95)00050-x.

5. Mayo Clinic, "Anorgasmia in Women: Symptoms and Causes," https://www.mayoclinic.org/diseases-conditions/anorgasmia/symptoms -causes/syc-20369422.

6. K. Wallen and E. A. Lloyd, "Female Sexual Arousal: Genital Anatomy and Orgasm in Intercourse," *Hormones and Behavior* 59, no. 5 (May 2011): 780–792, https://doi.org/10.1016/j.yhbeh.2010.12.004.

7. Harvard Health, "When an SSRI Medication Impacts Your Sex Life," https://www.health.harvard.edu/womens-health/when-an-ssri-medication -impacts-your-sex-life.

CHAPTER 7

1. Emily Nagoski, *Come As You Are: The Surprising New Science That Will Transform Your Sex Life* (New York: Simon & Schuster, 2015), 48–50.

2. Holly N. Thomas et al., "'I Want to Feel Like I Used to Feel': A Qualitative Study of Causes of Low Libido in Postmenopausal Women," *Menopause* 27, no. 3 (March 2020): 289–294, https://www.nhs.uk/conditions/loss-of -libido, https://doi.org/10.1097/GME.0000000000001455; C. R. Emerson, "Review of Low Libido in Women," *International Journal of STD & AIDS* 21, no 5 (May 2010): 312–316, https://doi.org/10.1258/ijsa.2010.009461.

3. Rosemary Basson, "The Female Sexual Response: A Different Model," *Journal of Sex & Marital Therapy* 26, no. 1 (February 2000): 51–65, https://doi.org/10.1080/009262300278641.

4. William H. Masters and Virginia E. Johnson, *Human Sexual Response* (New York: Little Brown, 1966).

5. R. Basson, "Testosterone Therapy for Reduced Libido in Women," *Therapeutic Advances in Endocrinology and Metabolism* 1, no. 4 (2010): 155164, https://doi.org/10.1177/ 2042018810379588.

6. R. Krysiak et al., "Sexual Function and Depressive Symptoms in Young Women with Elevated Macroprolactin Content: A Pilot Study," *Endocrine* 53 (February 2016): 291–298, https://doi.org/10.1007/s12020-016-0898-5.

CHAPTER 9

1. L. T. Gettler, "Longitudinal Evidence That Fatherhood Decreases Testosterone in Human Males," *Proceedings of the National Academy of Sciences of the United States of America* 108, no. 39 (September 2011): 16194–16199, https://doi.org/10.1073/pnas.1105403108.

CHAPTER 10

1. FDA, "Menopause," https://www.fda.gov/consumers/womens-health -topics/menopause.

2. R. F. Baumeister, K. R. Catanese, and K. D. Vohs, "Is There a Gender Difference in Strength of Sex Drive? Theoretical Views, Conceptual Distinctions, and a Review of Relevant Evidence," *Personality and Social Psychology Review* 5, no. 3 (2001), 242–273, https://doi.org/10.1207/S153 27957PSPR0503_5.

3. Susan R. Davis and Jane Tran, "Testosterone Influences Libido and Well Being in Women," *Trends in Endocrinology & Metabolism* 12, no. 1 (2001), 33–37, https://doi.org/10.1016/S1043-2760(00)00333-7. See also S. M. van Anders, "Testosterone and Sexual Desire in Healthy Women and Men," *Archives of Sexual Behavior* 41 (2012): 1471–1484, https://doi .org/10.1007/s10508-012-9946-2.

4. B. Zumoff et al., "Twenty-Four-Hour Mean Plasma Testosterone Concentration Declines with Age in Normal Premenopausal Women," *Journal of Clinical Endocrinology & Metabolism* 80, no. 4 (1995): 1429–1430, https://doi.org/10.1210/jcem.80.4.7714119.

5. Jean A. King et al., "Association of Stress, Hostility and Plasma Testosterone Levels," *Neuroendocrinology Letters* 26, no. 4 (2005): 355– 360, https://pdfs.semanticscholar.org/cbe3/7fc7717ff2e1e02cdbcfe3f60d6 1867c6cda.pdf.

6. Andrew T. Goldstein et al., "Polymorphisms of the Androgen Receptor Gene and Hormonal Contraceptive Induced Provoked Vestibulodynia," *Journal of Sexual Medicine* 11, no. 11 (November 2014), 2764–2771, https://doi.org/10.1111/jsm.12668.

7. R. V. Clark et al., "Large Divergence in Testosterone Concentrations Between Men and Women: Frame of Reference for Elite Athletes in Sex-Specific Competition in Sports: A Narrative Review," *Clinical Endocrinology* 90, no. 1 (2019): 15–22, https://doi.org/10.1111/cen.13840.

8. K. L. See, M. See, and C. Gluud, "Liver Pathology Associated with the Use of Anabolic-Androgenic Steroids," *Liver International* 12, no. 2 (1992): 73–79, https://doi.org/10.1111/j.1600 0676.1992.tb00560.x.

9. L. R. Nelson and S. E. Bulun, "Estrogen Production and Action," *Journal of the American Academy of Dermatology* 45, no. 3 (2001): S116–S124, https://doi.org/10.1067/mjd.2001.117432.

10. S. Gandy, "Estrogen and Neurodegeneration," *Neurochemical Research* 28, no. 7 (2003): 1003–1008, https://doi.org/10.1023/a:1023246921127.

11. J. A. E. Manson et al., "The Women's Health Initiative Hormone Therapy Trials: Update and Overview of Health Outcomes During the Intervention and Post-Stopping Phases," *JAMA* 310, no. 13 (2003): 1353–1368, https://doi.org/10.1001/jama.2013.278040.

12. R. C. Travis and T. J. Key, "Oestrogen Exposure and Breast Cancer Risk," *Breast Cancer Research* 5, no. 5 (2003): 239–247, https://doi.org/10.1186/bcr628.

13. "Estrogen Hormone Therapy Inhibits Alzheimer's Gene," http://www.alzheimersweekly.com/2013/02/estrogen-hormone-therapy-inhibits.html; A. Berent-Spillson et al., "Distinct Cognitive Effects of Estrogen and Progesterone in Menopausal Women," *Psychoneuroendocrinology* 59 (2015): 25–36, https://doi.org/10.1016/j.psyneuen.2015.04.020.

14. S. Chaikittisilpa, K. Soimongkol, and U. Jaisamrarn, "Efficacy of Oral Estrogen Plus Testosterone Gel to Improve Sexual Function in Postmenopausal Women," *Climacteric* 22, no. 5 (2019): 460–465, https://doi.org/10.1080/13697137.2019.1577378.

15. A. C. Rodriguez et al., "Estrogen Signaling in Endometrial Cancer: A Key Oncogenic Pathway with Several Open Questions," *Hormones and Cancer* 10, nos. 2–3 (2019): 51–63, https://doi.org/10.1007/s12672-019-0358-9.

16. N. Magon and S. Kalra, "The Orgasmic History of Oxytocin: Love, Lust, and Labor," *Indian Journal of Endocrinology and Metabolism* 15, suppl. 3 (2011): S156–S161, https://doi.org/10.4103/2230-8210.84851.

17. Marinus H. Van IJzendoorn, and Marian J. Bakermans-Kranenburg, "A Sniff of Trust: Meta-analysis of the Effects of Intranasal Oxytocin Administration on Face Recognition, Trust to In-Group, and Trust to Out-Group," *Psychoneuroendocrinology* 62 (December 2015): 180–188, https://doi.org/10.1016/j.psyneuen.2011.07.008.

18. L. M. Tracy et al., "Oxytocin and the Modulation of Pain Experience: Implications for Chronic Pain Management," *Neuroscience & Biobehavioral*

Reviews 55 (2015): 53–67, https://doi.org/10.1016/j.neubiorev.2015.04.013; F. Mancini et al., "Pain Relief by Touch: A Quantitative Approach," *Pain* 155, no. 3 (2014): 635–642, https://doi.org/10.1016/j.pain.2013.12.024.

CHAPTER 11

1. R. Baid and R. Agarwal, "Flibanserin: A Controversial Drug for Female Hypoactive Sexual Desire Disorder," *Industrial Psychiatry Journal* 27, no. 1 (2018): 154–157, https://doi.org/10.4103/ipj.ipj_20_16.

2. Conflicting info: FDA, "Highlights of Prescribing Information," https://www.accessdata.fda.gov/drugsatfda_docs/label/2017/020379 s032lbl.pdf; Lawrence Altman, "F.D.A. Approves an Injection to Treat Sexual Impotence," *New York Times*, July 8, 1995, https://www.nytimes .com/1995/07/08/us/fda-approves-an-injection-to-treat-sexual -impotence.html; U.S. Food and Drug Administration; National Drug Code Directory: Caverject, 2019, https://www.accessdata.fda.gov/scripts /cder/ndc/dsp_searchresult.cfm.

3. Viagra was first approved in 1998: US Food and Drug Administration, Drug Approvals and Databases, 1998, https://www.accessdata.fda .gov/drugsatfda_docs/NDA/98/viagra/viagra_toc.cfm.

4. A. Holdcroft, "Gender Bias in Research: How Does It Affect Evidence Based Medicine?" *Journal of the Royal Society of Medicine* 100, no. 1 (2007): 2–3, https://doi.org/10.1177/014107680710000102.

5. S. M. Stahl et al., "A Review of the Neuropharmacology of Bupropion, a Dual Norepinephrine and Dopamine Reuptake Inhibitor," *Primary Care Companion to the Journal of Clinical Psychiatry* 6, no. 4 (2004): 159–166, https://doi.org/10.4088/pcc.v06n0403.

6. Asher Mullard, "FDA Approves Female Sexual Dysfunction Drug," *Nature Reviews Drug Discovery* 14, no. 10 (October 1, 2015): 669, https:// doi.org/10.1038/nrd4757. PMID 26424353.

7. Andrew Pollack, "FDA Approves Addyi, a Libido Pill for Women," *New York Times*, August 18, 2015, retrieved September 13, 2019, https:// www.nytimes.com/2015/08/19/business/fda-approval-addyi-female -viagra.html; Harry Holt and Jeffrey Tingen, "Flibanserin (Addyi) for Hypoactive Sexual Desire Disorder in Premenopausal Women," *American*

Family Physician 93, no. 10 (May 2015): 826–828, https://www.aafp.org /afp/2016/0515/p826.html.

8. FDA, "FDA Approves New Treatment for Hypoactive Sexual Desire Disorder in Premenopausal Women," June 19, 2018 [press release], https:// www.fda.gov/news-events/press-announcements/fda-approves-new -treatment-hypoactive-sexual-desire-disorder-premenopausal-women.

9. D. Franic, Z. Iternička, and M. Franić-Ivanišević, "Platelet-Rich Plasma (PRP) for the Treatment of Vulvar Lichen Sclerosus in a Premenopausal Woman: A Case Report," *Case Reports in Women's Health* 18 (2018): e00062, ISSN 2214-9112, https://doi.org/10.1016/j.crwh.2018.e00062.

10. T. E. Foster et al., "Platelet-Rich Plasma: From Basic Science to Clinical Applications," *American Journal of Sports Medicine* 37, no. 11 (2009): 2259–2272, https://doi.org/10.1177/0363546509349921.

11. C. Runels et al., "A Pilot Study of the Effect of Localized Injections of Autologous Platelet Rich Plasma (PRP) for the Treatment of Female Sexual Dysfunction," *Journal of Women's Health Care* 3 (2014): 169, https:// doi.org/10.4172/2167-0420.1000169.

12. A. Higgins, M. Nash, and A. M. Lynch, "Antidepressant-Associated Sexual Dysfunction: Impact, Effects, and Treatment," *Drug, Healthcare and Patient Safety* 2 (2010): 141–150, https://doi.org/10.2147/DHPS.S7634.

CHAPTER 12

1. T. Landry et al., "The Treatment of Provoked Vestibulodynia: A Critical Review," *Clinical Journal of Pain* 24 (2008): 155–171.

CHAPTER 13

1. Cheryl Karcher and Neil Sadick, "Vaginal Rejuvenation Using Energy-Based Devices," *International Journal of Women's Dermatology* 2, no. 3 (2016): 85–88, ISSN 2352-6475, https://doi.org/10.1016/j .ijwd.2016.05.003.

2. M. B. MacBride, D. J. Rhodes, and L. T. Shuster, "Vulvovaginal Atrophy," *Mayo Clinic Proceedings* 85, no. 1 (2010): 87–94. https://doi.org/ doi:10.4065/mcp.2009.0413.

3. M. Fidela et al., "A Randomized Clinical Trial Comparing Vaginal Laser Therapy to Vaginal Estrogen Therapy in Women with Genitourinary Syndrome of Menopause: The VeLVET Trial," *Menopause* 27, no. 1 (January 2020): 50–56, https://doi.org/10.1097/GME.0000000000001416.

4. C. Arroyo, "Fractional CO_2 Laser Treatment for Vulvovaginal Atrophy Symptoms and Vaginal Rejuvenation in Perimenopausal Women," *International Journal of Women's Health* 9 (2017): 591–595, https://doi.org/10.2147/IJWH.S136857.

5. In 2017, Jeanne Scheele of the Kaplan Center for Integrative Medicine tested the effectiveness of cold laser therapy, using the ML830 laser, on twenty-two Kaplan Center patients who presented with pelvic pain. The results point to significant and consistent improvement. Treatments by Kaplan Center, October 9, 2017, "Cold Laser Therapy for Treating Pelvic Pain," https://kaplanclinic.com/cold-laser-therapy-for-pelvic-pain/.

6. A. Lev-Sagie, A. Kopitman, and A. Brzezinski, "Low-Level Laser Therapy for the Treatment of Provoked Vestibulodynia—A Randomized, Placebo-Controlled Pilot Trial," *Journal of Sexual Medicine* 14, no. 11 (2017): 1403–1411.

7. On vaginal "tightening" and laxity: S. Lalji and P. Lozanova, "Evaluation of the Safety and Efficacy of a Monopolar Nonablative Radiofrequency Device for the Improvement of Vulvo-Vaginal Laxity and Urinary Incontinence," *Journal of Cosmetic Dermatology* 16 (2017): 230–234, https://doi.org/10.1111/jocd.12348. On sensation and orgasm: R. M. Alinsod, "Transcutaneous Temperature Controlled Radiofrequency for Orgasmic Dysfunction," *Lasers in Surgery and Medicine* 48, 7 (2016): 641–645, https://doi.org/10.1002/lsm.22537.

CHAPTER 14

1. B. Marcus, "Changes in a Woman's Sexual Experience and Expectations Following the Introduction of Electric Vibrator Assistance," *International Society for Sexual Medicine* (2010), https://doi.org/10.1111/j.1743-6109.2010.02132.x.

CHAPTER 15

1. Dorothy Tennov, *Love and Limerence: The Experience of Being in Love* (New York: Scarborough House, 1999).

2. Theresa L. Crenshaw, *The Alchemy of Love and Lust* (New York: Simon and Schuster, 1996).

3. Helen Fisher, *Why We Love: The Nature and Chemistry of Romantic Love* (New York: Henry Holt and Company, 2004).

4. Wednesday Martin, "The Bored Sex," *Atlantic*, February 14, 2019.

5. Esther Perel, *Mating in Captivity: Unlocking Erotic Intelligence* (New York: HarperCollins, 2006).

CHAPTER 16

1. Andrew Octavian Asmita, Joshua Kuruvilla, and Anna Pick Kiong Ling, "Harnessing Neuroplasticity: Modern Approaches and Clinical Future," *International Journal of Neuroscience* 128, no. 11 (May 14, 2018): 1061–1077, https://doi.org/10.1080/00207454.2018.1466781, ISSN 1563-5279. PMID 29667473.

2. Sebastian J. Lipina and Jorge A. Colombo, *Poverty and Brain Development During Childhood: An Approach from Cognitive Psychology and Neuroscience* (Washington, DC: American Psychological Association, 2009).

3. Bryan Kolb and Ian Q. Whishaw, *Fundamentals of Human Neuropsychology*, 5th ed. (New York: Worth Publishers, 2003).

4. A. B. Losecaat Vermeer, I. Riečanský, and C. Eisenegger, Chapter 9: "Competition, Testosterone, and Adult Neurobehavioral Plasticity," edited by Bettina Studer and Stefan Knecht, *Progress in Brain Research* 229 (2016): 213–238, https://doi.org/10.1016/bs.pbr.2016.05.004/.

5. B. Leuner, E. R. Glasper, and E. Gould, "Sexual Experience Promotes Adult Neurogenesis in the Hippocampus Despite an Initial Elevation in Stress Hormones," *PLoS ONE* 5, no. 7 (2010): e11597, https://doi.org/10.1371/journal.pone.0011597.

6. M. Bangert and E. O. Altenmüller, "Mapping Perception to Action in Piano Practice: A Longitudinal DC-EEG Study. *BMC Neuroscience* 4, no. 26 (2003), https://doi.org/10.1186/1471-2202-4-26.

7. L. D. Hamilton, E. A. Fogle, and C. M. Meston, "The Roles of Testosterone and Alpha-Amylase in Exercise-Induced Sexual Arousal in Women," *Journal of Sexual Medicine* 5, no. 4 (2008): 845–853, https://doi .org/10.1111/j.1743-6109.2007.00751.x.

8. J. Money, "Paraphilias: Phenomenology and Classification," *American Journal of Psychotherapy* 38, no. 2 (April 1984): 164–179, https://doi .org/10.1176/appi.psychotherapy.1984.38.2.164; John Money, *Lovemaps: Clinical Concepts of Sexual/Erotic Health and Pathology, Paraphilia, and Gender Transposition in Childhood, Adolescence, and Maturity* (New York: Prometheus Books, 1986).

CHAPTER 17

1. Jack Morin, *The Erotic Mind: Unlocking the Inner Sources of Passion and Fulfillment* (New York: HarperCollins, 1995).

2. Daniel Bergner, *What Do Women Want? Adventures in the Science of Female Desire* (Edinburgh, Scotland: Canongate Books, 2013).

3. Ogi Ogas and Sai Gaddam, *A Billion Wicked Thoughts: What the World's Largest Experiment Reveals About Human Desire* (New York: Plume, 2012), 106.

4. Ogas and Gaddam, *A Billion Wicked Thoughts*, 221.

5. Anthony Cox and Maryanne Fisher, "The Texas Billionaire's Pregnant Bride: An Evolutionary Interpretation of Romance Fiction Titles," *Journal of Social, Evolutionary, and Cultural Psychology* 3, no. 4 (2009), 386–401.

6. Ogas and Gaddam, *A Billion Wicked Thoughts*, 101; Matthew Philips, "The Neuroscience Behind Sexual Desire: Authors of A Billion Wicked Thoughts Answer Your Questions" [blog], posted May 17, 2011, https:// freakonomics.com/2011/05/17/the-neuroscience-behind-sexual-desire -authors-of-a-billion-wicked-thoughts-answer-your-questions/.

7. Alan Shindel and Charles A. Moser, "Why Are the Paraphilias Mental Disorders" *Journal of Sexual Medicine* 8, no. 3 (2011): 927–929.

8. Morin, *The Erotic Mind*, 128.

ACKNOWLEDGMENTS

With sincere gratitude:

Michael Werner, without you this book simply would not exist. You used the 100-point model to illustrate the complexity of infertility to me, and that ultimately formed the basis of my thinking about women's sexuality. We've had an extraordinary working relationship for twenty years: your guts and business acumen, as well as our shared planning, laughing, arguing, and learning, are what have allowed us to embark on this crazy venture called Maze Health.

While on the subject of Maze Women's Health: Melissa Ferrara, you reviewed all of the medical parts of this book more times than I'd like to count. Thank you. More importantly, thank you for years of commitment to your patients and passion for women's sexual health. Helen Leff, your thoughtful readings and suggestions were so helpful. Melissa, Helen, Jackie Giannelli, and Jennifer Dembo, our patients are the beneficiaries of your staunch advocacy. I truly believe the world is a better place because of what we do. Tammy Williams, Amanda Cavuto, and Sue Bernard, you make the office a place where we can all laugh and where we want to be every day. That's not easy, and I hope you know how much I cherish it. Thank you.

Wendy Sherman, how did I happen to stumble upon the world's best agent? You do so much: advising, suggesting, covering for my gaffes, and just being an all-around "fairy godmother." I just want you to know how blessed I feel to have met you.

Callie Deitrick, thank you for rescuing me from the slush pile. I can't wait to see your first book, because I know the illustrations will capture who you truly are: caring, competent, and generous of spirit.

To the whole team at Hachette: Renee Sedliar, for your calm, sensible, gentle but firm correctives, thank you from the bottom of this first-time author's heart. I went into this nervous and couldn't have asked for a kinder, more thoughtful editor. Mary Ann Naples, you believed in this project from its inception and nothing could have made me happier. Alison Dalafave, thank you for always being there picking up all the pieces the rest of us missed. And thanks to Fred Francis and Iris Bass for cleaning up all of the extraneous "ands" and "sos." It was not an easy job. Lauren Rosenthal, thank you for holding up the PR, and Elizabeth Belsky, thanks for the ongoing advice. Who knew social media was marketing?

Thanks to the whole SoulCamp Team: Michelle Goldblum, Alexandra Hampton, Alison Leipzig, Hanna Coward, and Jess Manuszak. You made a terribly overwhelming job lively and fun and always hopping. Richelle Fredson, you got me started Instagramming on my pink hat and the rest is history. Jazzie Morgan, what can I say? Everyone needs a social media "jazzie." "k'shma keyn hi" I'm glad we found each other. Thank you all!

To all the young women who proofread for me along the way, I hope you learned something. I certainly learned how bad my grammar was: Shoshana Benjamin, my amazing daughter-in-law Daniella Penn, and Channa Fisch.

Special shout-out to Amy Gamerman. We still have a book in our future, but your encouragement and thoughtfulness helped guide my thinking. And, David Wohlsifer, thanks for the last-minute neuroplasticity read-through. You know how much your opinion and friendship mean.

To my family: Yedidya, Yishai, and Shalhevet, although you are not around these days, I hope you realize that I still have all of you sitting on my shoulder making wry comments as I write. I'm waiting with bated breath for your, no doubt, significantly more intellectual books and truly hope this one doesn't embarrass you all too much.

Elliot, when I was in the last months of pregnancy and couldn't make it up the hills, you would put your hand on my back to give me the extra push I needed. That pretty much sums up our relationship. I come up with more projects and ideas than are practical (or even possible). But you are always, always there believing in me, supporting me, and helping me get that last push when I inevitably run out of steam. This project was no different. I love you.

INDEX